W0106385

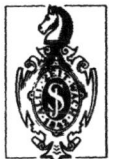

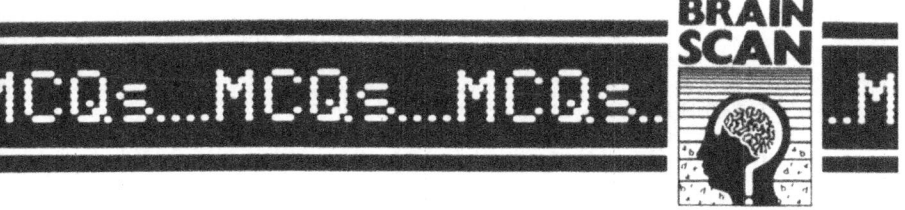

Philip Helliwell · Howard Bird · Verna Wrigh

Rheumatology

Springer-Verlag
London Berlin Heidelberg New York
Paris Tokyo

Philip S. Helliwell, MA, DM, MRCP
Research Fellow, University of Leeds, Rheumatism and Rehabilitation Research Unit,
University of Leeds, 36, Clarendon Road, Leeds LS2 9PJ

Howard A. Bird, MD, FRCP
Senior Lecturer in Rheumatology, University of Leeds,
Consultant Rheumatologist General Infirmary at Leeds and
Royal Bath Hospital, Harrogate HG1 2PS

Verna Wright, MD, FRCP
ARC Professor of Rheumatology, Rheumatism and Rehabilitation Research Unit,
University of Leeds, 36 Clarendon Road, Leeds LS2 9PJ

Publishers note: the 'Brainscan' logo is reproduced by courtesy of The Editor,
Geriatric Medicine, Modern Medicine GB Ltd

ISBN-13:978-3-540-19554-2   e-ISBN-13:978-1-4471-1691-2
DOI: 10.1007/978-1-4471-1691-2

British Library Cataloguing in Publication Data
Helliwell, Philip, 1947–   Rheumatology.   1. Man. Rheumatic diseases
I. Title   II. Bird, Howard, 1945–   III. Wright, V. (Verna)   616.7′23
ISBN-13:978-3-540-19554-2

Library of Congress Cataloging-in-Publication Data
Helliwell, Philip, 1947–
Rheumatology/Philip Helliwell, Howard Bird, Verna Wright.
p.   cm. — (Brainscan MCQ's)   Includes bibliographies and index.
ISBN-13:978-3-540-19554-2
1. Rheumatology—Examinations, questions, etc. I. Bird, H. A.
(Howard Anthony), 1945–   . II. Wright, Verna. III. Title.   IV. Series.
[DNLM: 1. Rheumatology—examination questions.   WE 18 H477r]
RC952.H45   1989   616.7′23′076—dc20   DNLM/DLC
for Library of Congress   89-6136
                                                                        CIP

Filmset by Macmillan India Ltd., Bangalore 560025

2128/3916–543210 (Printed on acid-free paper)

Preface

This selection of MCQs in rheumatology is largely aimed at MRCP candidates but some will be difficult for established rheumatologists and some will be possible for enthusiastic medical students. The format of the questions largely follows that used in the MRCP Part I examination with a few exceptions employing diagrams and assertion/reason questions (these are explained on p. vi). No guidance on scoring is included since we feel that if an honest attempt is made at answering the question then the process is, in itself, educational. Some of the answers have been determined only after considerable discussion between us and as far as possible we have attempted to convey the views expressed in accepted British texts. Where answers seem contentious an appropriate reference has been given. Similarly the layout of the chapters largely follows that adopted by standard text books although the basic sciences have been incorporated within the individual chapters.

We wish to thank Mrs. Dora Smith for typing and re-typing the manuscript according to the foibles of three different authors.

Leeds, October 1988
P. S. Helliwell
H. A. Bird
V. Wright

Assertion/Reason Questions

These questions consist of two statements. The first statement is numbered 1 and the second is numbered 2. For example:

1. A positive family history of ankylosing spondylitis (AS) is often found in patients with this disease.
2. There is an increased incidence of HLA-B27 antigen in patients with AS.

Before selecting the correct key you have to answer two or sometimes three questions.

1. Is the first statement on its own a true or false statement? In the example given, AS does run in families. Answer, True.
2. Is the second statement on its own a true or false statement? In the example given, there is an increased incidence of HLA-B27 in patients with AS. Answer, True.

If either of these statements is false, the correct key will be c, d or e (see the code which follows). If both statements are true, you have to answer the third question:

3. Is the second statement a correct explanation of the first statement? In the example given, the answer is "Yes", B27 is probably a susceptibility gene to AS. Answer, a.

The code for answering these questions is as follows:

a. If both statements are true and the second statement is a correct explanation of the first statement.
b. If both statements are true but the second statement is not a correct explanation of the first statement.
c. If the first statement is true but the second statement is false.
d. If the first statement is false but the second statement is true.
e. If both statements are false.

These instructions will be summarised where the questions appear.

Contents

1. Rheumatoid Arthritis

Q.1.1 In rheumatoid arthritis

a. the majority of subjects have a positive sheep cell agglutination test in a titre of 1 in 32 or more
b. 25% of subjects have a positive anti-nuclear factor by direct immunofluorescence
c. the autoantibody responsible for a positive sheep cell agglutination test belongs to the IgG class of immunoglobulin
d. autoantibodies to thyroid microsomes and gastric parietal cells are commonly found but are rarely of pathogenic significance
e. autoantibody production results directly from the presence of Class 2 MHC antigen DR4

Q.1.2 Subcutaneous rheumatoid nodules

a. are most frequently found on the extensor surface of the elbow
b. often have a necrotic centre
c. are almost invariably associated with high titres of IgM rheumatoid factor
d. may, when in tendon sheaths, be mistaken for xanthomata
e. may involute in response to treatment with disease-modifying drugs

For answers see over

Answers

A.1.1 a. T—85% have a positive latex test.
      b. T—Usually more common in females. The figure quoted for males is 14%.
      c. F—The antibody responsible for sheep cell agglutination is classically an IgM, but IgG and IgA antibodies have been described.
      d. F—There is an association between other autoimmune disorders and rheumatoid arthritis.
      e. F—DR4 is found more often in Europeans with RA but no HLA antigen is specifically associated with autoantibody production.

A.1.2 a. T—Other sites where they may occur are the scalp, sclera, abdominal wall, peritoneum, heart and pericardium.
      b. T—With characteristic pallisading histiocytes around the centre.
      c. T—In over 95% of cases nodularity is associated with seropositivity although in a small percentage of cases classical rheumatoid factor may be absent.
      d. T
      e. T

Q.1.3 The following statements are true of a 48-year-old male with active seropositive nodular rheumatoid arthritis presenting in Casualty with anterior chest pains. The ECG in the figures is recorded:

  a. The patient should be treated as a case of acute myocardial infarction
  b. High dose oral steroids should be commenced
  c. Subsequent evaluation should include an echocardiogram
  d. Urea and electrolytes should be checked
  e. ANF should be checked

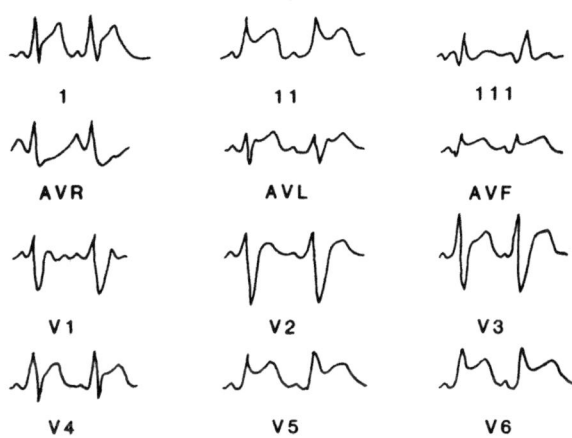

Q.1.4 The pulmonary complications of rheumatoid arthritis include

  a. pleural effusion
  b. pleural calcification
  c. pulmonary fibrosis (fibrosing alveolitis)
  d. pulmonary hypertension
  e. haemoptysis
  f. hoarseness

For answers see over

Answers

A.1.3 a. F—The ECG shows widespread coved ST segments indicative of acute pericarditis.

      b. T—This may help.

      c. T—Since a pericardial effusion may subsequently develop.

      d. T—Since other causes such as uraemia may be found.

      e. F—There is no evidence that ANF positively influences the development of pericarditis in classical rheumatoid arthritis.

A.1.4 a. T—This may occasionally be the first manifestation of rheumatoid arthritis.

      b. F—Pleural calcification is more often seen in asbestosis. Peripheral pulmonary nodules, seen in rheumatoid arthritis, may occasionally mimic pleural disease.

      c. T

      d. T—Although pulmonary hypertension is more usually seen in connective tissue diseases, pulmonary artery involvement in rheumatoid arthritis may occur especially in association with Raynaud's phenomenon.

      e. F

      f. T—This may be due to arthritis of the cricoarytenoid joints.

Q.1.5 In rheumatoid arthritis, a hyperviscosity syndrome due to elevated plasma proteins may occur. Invariably this is associated with a high titre of rheumatoid factor. The following clinical features may be present:

a. Dyspnoea
b. Dizziness
c. Diplopia
d. Skin haemorrhage
e. Paraesthesiae

Q.1.6 In the treatment of rheumatoid arthritis

a. the symptomatic benefit from non-steroidal anti-inflammatory drugs is associated with a decrease in the ESR and level of C-reactive protein in the blood
b. gold injections modify the course of the disease
c. some side-effects to D-penicillamine and gold may be predicted on a genetic basis
d. plasmapheresis is helpful in treatment
e. steroids predispose patients to septic arthritis

Q.1.7 A 32-year-old active female with known rheumatoid arthritis develops an acutely painful calf. The following statements are true:

a. She should be treated with bedrest and anti-coagulants until a firm diagnosis is established
b. A positive Homan's sign helps
c. Pain starting behind the knee joint is important
d. An ascending venogram is the investigation of choice
e. Bruising around the ankle may be helpful

For answers see over

Answers

A.1.5   a. T
  b. T
  c. T
  d. T
  e. T

In addition, the fundi may show blot haemorrhages and soft exudates and, in extreme cases, papilloedema. There is often a markedly raised plasma viscosity (often greater than 2.0).

A.1.6   a. F—The improvement with non-steroidal anti-inflammatory drugs is not reflected in a decrease in the inflammatory indices. These fall on treatment with disease-modifying drugs.
  b. T
  c. T—Patients with HLA DR3 are more susceptible to nephrotoxic side-effects of these drugs.
  d. F—Although theoretically this should help in systemic vasculitis in rheumatoid arthritis, where presumably immune complexes are involved.
  e. F—Patients with rheumatoid arthritis are prone to septic arthritis; steroids mask the presence of septic arthritis.

A.1.7   a. F
  b. F
  c. T
  d. F
  e. T

Pain in the calf in a patient with arthritis should arouse suspicion of a ruptured Baker's (popliteal) cyst. Pain starting behind the knee with subsequent bruising around the ankle are helpful signs. If in doubt a less traumatic investigation is a contrast arthrogram to outline the leaking popliteal cyst.

Q.1.8 **The following may be manifestations of rheumatoid arthritis:**

  a. Erythema multiforme
  b. Erythema nodosum
  c. Solitary pulmonary granuloma
  d. Recurrent iritis
  e. Amyloidosis
  f. Peripheral neuropathy

Q.1.9 **The following pathological features on synovial biopsy are diagnostic of rheumatoid arthritis:**

  a. Fibrinous exudate
  b. An infiltrate of lymphocytes and plasma cells
  c. The presence of many polymorphonuclear leucocytes
  d. The presence of lymphoid follicles
  e. Multinucleate giant cells
  f. All of the above
  g. None of the above

Q.1.10 **The following symptoms and signs are of value in the early diagnosis of rheumatoid arthritis:**

  a. Symptoms worse in the early morning
  b. Heel pain
  c. Weakness of grip
  d. Ulnar deviation
  e. Subcutaneous nodules on the ulnar border of the forearm
  f. Fusiform swelling of the proximal interphalangeal joints

For answers see over

Answers

A.1.8 a. F—Unless as a reaction to drugs such as sulphasalazine.
   b. F—Erythema nodosum from whatever cause may be associated with synovitis.
   c. T—As in Caplan's syndrome, which consists of pulmonary nodules in association with either rheumatoid arthritis or positive test for rheumatoid factor superimposed on a background of pneumoconiosis.
   d. F—Episcleritis and scleritis may occur in arthritis.
   e. T—If looked for on rectal biopsy, amyloid may be found in 13%–17% of cases of rheumatoid arthritis examined at postmortem in hospital, presumably after many years of disease.
   f. T—Usually due to vasculitis involving the vasa nervorum.

A.1.9 a. F
   b. F
   c. F
   d. F
   e. F
   f. F
   g. T

The specificity of histological findings in rheumatoid arthritis is extremely low and rarely helpful in diagnosis. The uncommon microscopic synovial granuloma is perhaps the only pathological lesion which is seen characteristically in rheumatoid arthritis.

A.1.10 a. T—Early morning stiffness is one of the cardinal symptoms and diagnostic features of rheumatoid arthritis.
   b. F—This is more common in seronegative spondarthritis.
   c. T—Often one of the first symptoms.
   d. F—Ulnar deviation usually occurs late in the disease as a result of chronic inflammation of the metacarpophalangeal joints.
   e. F—Nodules are usually a later manifestation although occasionally rheumatoid arthritis may present with subcutaneous nodules before any other symptoms and signs appear.
   f. T

Q.1.11   In the treatment of the patient with early severe rheumatoid arthritis the most important initial measures are

a. bed-rest
b. aspirin
c. joint splints
d. steroids
e. physiotherapy

Q.1.12   Rheumatoid arthritis and rheumatoid arteritis differ in a number of ways. The following features most closely relate to rheumatoid arteritis:

a. Reduced serum complement level
b. Immune complexes in synovial fluid
c. Dermal necrosis with ulcers
d. Episcleritis

Q.1.13   The most appropriate indication for instituting gold or other remittive therapy in rheumatoid arthritis is

a. rheumatoid titre greater than 1 in 1280
b. persistent pain in more than six joints despite the use of maximum tolerated doses of two non-steroidal anti-inflammatory drugs
c. persistent swelling at multiple joints despite the use of maximum tolerated doses of aspirin or of non-steroidal anti-inflammatory drugs over three months
d. rheumatoid nodules
e. subluxation at more than three joints on X-ray

For answers see over

Answers

A.1.11

	1968	*1988*
a.	T	F
b.	T	F
c.	T	T
d.	F	(T)
e.	F	T

This question exemplifies the changing trends in rheumatology. Importantly it emphasises the swing away from aspirin as a first-line drug in the UK (but not in the USA) and the emphasis now on keeping the patient active, even in acute arthritis. The answer for steroids is bracketed since in certain centres high dose intravenous methylprednisolone is currently used in cases of early severe rheumatoid arthritis.

A.1.12

a. T
b. F
c. T
d. T

In rheumatoid arteritis, immune complexes capable of consuming complement are found in the serum. The vasculitic ulcers which are often found on the lower limbs and are deep, penetrating and punched out in appearance, together with the episcleritis, are manifestations of ischaemia.

A.1.13

a. F
b. F
c. T
d. F
e. F

The usual indication for disease-modifying anti-rheumatic drugs is persistent synovitis in several joints. The joint inflammation should be objectively apparent and many would feel that the development of erosive changes are an indication.

Although rheumatoid nodules may shrink or even disappear on appropriate remittive treatment, this is not the usual indication for starting this therapy.

Q.1.14 Rheumatoid factor

    a. may be any class of immunoglobin
    b. may be present in chronic infections
    c. is detectable in a small percentage of healthy adults
    d. may promote the clearance of immune complexes by the reticulo-endothelial system
    e. in high titre is strongly predictive of bone erosions

Q.1.15 A 33-year-old white female with a history of joint pain and swelling is admitted to hospital. Her total blood count reveals a white blood count of 1300 per cu.mm. with the following differential: lymphocytes 90%, monocytes 5%, eosinophils 3%, polymorphs 2%. The most likely diagnosis is

    a. Felty's syndrome
    b. SLE
    c. rheumatoid vasculitis
    d. overlap syndrome
    e. all of the above

Q.1.16 In the radiology of rheumatoid arthritis

    a. juxta-articular osteoporosis may be the first radiological sign
    b. atlantoaxial subluxation is the usual cause of cervical myelopathy
    c. periostitis is commonly found
    d. rheumatoid nodules may give rise to soft tissue calcification
    e. a "pencil-in-cup" appearance is a characteristic finding

For answers see over

Answers

A.1.14   a.   T—But usually we test for IgM.

b.   T—For example, sub-acute bacterial endocarditis or pulmonary tuberculosis.

c.   T—The incidence of positive rheumatoid factor in healthy adults increases with age. These false positives may be diminished by using a more specific test such as an ELISA but at the expense of some loss of sensitivity.

d.   T—Rheumatoid factor may normally play a positive role in infections.

e.   T—It is also predictive of extra-articular manifestations and is an indicator of a worse prognosis in rheumatoid arthritis.

A.1.15   a.   T

b.   F

c.   F

d.   F

e.   F

Rheumatoid arthritis with hypersplenism (Felty's syndrome). SLE can cause a severe lymphopenia. Severe neutropenia may also occur in rheumatoid arthritis as a side-effect of treatment with drugs such as gold. In Felty's syndrome the cell line most usually affected by the hypersplenism is the polymorphonuclear leucocyte and severe neutropenia with the risk of bacterial infection may ensue.

A.1.16   a.   T—But these changes are reversible.

b.   T—Spondylolisthesis at lower cervical levels may also cause cervical myelopathy.

c.   F—Periostitis is more commonly seen in psoriatic arthritis, Reiter's disease and hypertrophic pulmonary osteoarthropathy.

d.   F—Calcification in nodular structures may be seen in gout and in systemic sclerosis.

e.   F—"Pencil-in-cup" appearance is usually seen in psoriatic arthritis where osteolysis occurs at the proximal half of the joint.

Q.1.17 **The following clinical sign may be found in the eye in rheumatoid arthritis:**

a. Iritis
b. Episcleritis
c. Choroidoretinitis
d. Cataract
e. Maculopathy in subjects treated with chloroquine
f. Diplopia in subjects treated with penicillamine

Q.1.18 **In the rheumatoid hand**

a. there may be wasting of the thenar eminence
b. palmar erythema occurs
c. erosion of the distal interphalangeal joints on X-ray examination is common
d. ulnar deviation is due to attrition of the ulnar collateral ligament of the metacarpophalangeal joint
e. swan neck deformity is due to weakness of the dorsal interossei
f. rheumatoid nodules in the flexor tendon sheaths often cause "triggering" of the finger

Q.1.19 **In rheumatoid arthritis early interstitial lung fibrosis is characterised by**

a. cyanosis at rest
b. decreased ventilatory capacity
c. decreased FEV_1/FVC
d. bilateral reticular shadowing on chest X-ray
e. decreased pulmonary diffusing capacity

For answers see over

Answers

A.1.17 a. F—Iritis is seen in seronegative spondarthritis.
b. T—Although scleritis is more important and may ultimately lead to blindness due to involvement of the whole uveal tract.
c. F—This is more often seen associated with vasculitis in Behçet's disease.
d. T—When chronic steroid treatment has been administered.
e. T—Fundoscopy is necessary pre-treatment with chloroquine or related compounds and 6-monthly check-ups with fundoscopy, Ishihara colour vision testing, and visual acuity testing are required. Some ophthalmologists recommend electroretinograms at 6-monthly intervals also.
f. T—This may be the first symptom of penicillamine-induced myasthenic syndrome.

A.1.18 a. T—Carpal tunnel syndrome is common in rheumatoid arthritis due to compression of the median nerve in the carpal tunnel by inflammatory synovial tissue.
b. T—Other causes are pregnancy and cirrhosis.
c. F—Rheumatoid arthritis commonly affects the proximal interphalangeal and metacarpophalangeal joints. Distal interphalangeal joint erosions occasionally occur in osteoarthritis but more commonly occur due to psoriatic arthritis.
d. F—Ulnar deviation is thought to be due to the interplay of a number of factors, including attrition of the medial (i.e., radial) collateral ligament, the geometry of the metacarpophalangeal joint, and the direction of pull of the strong flexor tendons.
e. F—Swan neck deformity occurs due to tightening of the retinacular ligament across the proximal interphalangeal joint in conjunction with tightening of the intrinsic musculature of the hand. The resulting hyperextension of the proximal interphalangeal joint compromises the function of the extensor tendon.
f. F—More often triggering of the finger is due to narrowing of the internal diameter of the flexor tendon sheath due to inflammatory synovitis.

A.1.19 a. F—Rarely in early disease is there cyanosis at rest but the P_{O_2} may fall on exercise.
b. T
c. F—There is a restrictive defect but not an obstructive pattern.
d. T
e. T

Q.1.20 **A patient with rheumatoid arthritis is found to be anaemic. The following statements are appropriate:**

    a. Serum ferritin is a useful indicator of iron stores

    b. Hypochromia and microcytosis will respond to iron

    c. Faecal occult bloods are useful in determining the cause of the anaemia

    d. Where iron deficiency is confirmed, peptic ulceration is frequently found

    e. A normochromic normocytic blood film suggests that the anaemia is due to rheumatoid disease

Q.1.21 **In rheumatoid arthritis**

    a. asymptomatic pericarditis is frequently found

    b. myocarditis may occur

    c. mitral incompetence is a rare finding

    d. conduction defects may occur due to intra-cardiac rheumatoid nodules

    e. patients are protected from cardiovascular disease as a result of taking aspirin-like compounds

    f. all of the above are true

For answers see over

Answers

A.1.20 a. T—But caution is necessary since the serum ferritin is part of the acute phase response and generally an alternative, somewhat higher, lower limit of normal should be employed.

b. F—Defective iron utilisation and absorption occurs in rheumatoid arthritis, so that as the disease is treated iron is released for utilisation and the apparent iron-deficient picture is corrected.

c. F—There are a number of causes of false-positive faecal occult bloods. Furthermore, drug therapy with non-steroidal antiinflammatory drugs may cause positive faecal occult bloods because of gastric erosions or small bowel inflammation. Considering the unpleasantness of this investigation to the patient, the nursing staff and the laboratory, there is a poor yield of diagnostic information.

d. T—Up to 40% of patients with rheumatoid arthritis on treatment will have peptic ulceration although only a small percentage of these will have iron deficiency anaemia due to blood loss from these ulcers.

e. T

A.1.21 a. T—Up to 30% of cases at post-mortem and on ultrasound examination show evidence of pericardial inflammation.

b. F—Polymyositis may occur in skeletal muscle: some authorities have used electromyographic evidence to suggest this occurs in up to 30% of cases of rheumatoid arthritis. The cardiac muscle may be infiltrated by amyloid and myocardial infarction may occur due to coronary arteritis.

c. T—Due to granulomatous involvement of mitral valve.

d. T

e. F—Mortality data show patients with rheumatoid arthritis have a reduced life expectancy and this includes death due to coronary heart disease.

f. F

Q.1.22　A 50-year-old female is referred by her general practitioner following the discovery of abnormal liver function tests. She has a 10-year history of seropositive nodular rheumatoid arthritis and is established on treatment with sulphasalazine 2 g daily. The full blood count is normal. The following statements are true:

　　　a. A raised serum alkaline phosphatase may be found in rheumatoid arthritis in the absence of liver or bone pathology

　　　b. Elevated transaminases may occasionally be due to treatment with sulphasalazine

　　　c. Hepatosplenomegaly may be due to amyloid, confirmation of which is best obtained by liver biopsy

　　　d. A search for anti-mitochondrial antibodies is indicated

　　　e. The patient is likely to have Felty's syndrome

Q.1.23　These statements are true of Caplan's syndrome:

　　　a. The syndrome may be present in the absence of rheumatoid arthritis

　　　b. The syndrome is always associated with a positive rheumatoid factor

　　　c. It is more common in men

　　　d. The histological appearance of the pulmonary nodule is similar to that of the peripheral nodule in rheumatoid arthritis

　　　e. All of the above

　　　f. None of the above

Q.1.24　The following statements apply in Felty's syndrome:

　　　a. More males than females have this syndrome

　　　b. The sheep cell agglutination test is invariably positive

　　　c. Recurrence of leucopenia may follow splenectomy

　　　d. Patients most frequently die of septic phenomena

　　　e. Steroids invariably improve the total white blood count

　　　f. Hepatosplenomegaly may occur

For answers see over

Answers

A.1.22 a. T—Serum alkaline phosphatase of hepatic origin is part of the acute phase response.

b. T—Sulphasalazine may cause elevation of the liver transaminases indicating that therapy should be withdrawn.

c. T—Hepatosplenomegaly may be due to amyloid and liver biopsy would help to confirm this. More usually the presence of amyloid is investigated by rectal or gingival biopsies which are easier and safer to perform.

d. T—There is an increased incidence of primary biliary cirrhosis in rheumatoid arthritis.

e. F—If Felty's syndrome was present, leucopenia would be likely.

A.1.23 a. T
b. T
c. T
d. T
e. T
f. F

Caplan's syndrome consists of nodular pulmonary opacities in a patient with rheumatoid arthritis or in a patient with minimal or no obvious clinical rheumatoid arthritis but with a positive test for rheumatoid factor. Other industrial dust diseases have been implicated. The radiological appearance is of nodular opacities against a background of pneumoconiosis.

A.1.24 a. T
b. T—These patients also have more severe disease and more associated Sjögren's syndrome.

c. T
d. T
e. F—Steroids may improve white blood count and anaemia but not invariably. Steroids may also contribute to the risk of infection in this syndrome.

f. T—The spleen may weigh up to one kilogram and hepatosplenomegaly is the hallmark of this syndrome. The liver often shows nodular regenerative hyperplasia and portal hypertension.

Q.1.25 **The following statements reasonably reflect the prognosis of rheumatoid arthritis after five years duration of the disease:**

    a. Total recovery in 30%, crippled in 70%

    b. No patient free of symptoms, moderate loss of function in 40%, total loss in 60%

    c. About 10% practically free of symptoms, 80% moderately impaired, 10% severely impaired

    d. No patient free of symptoms, no patient severely impaired

    e. 50% free of symptoms, 50% impaired

For answers see over

Answers

A.1.25 a. F
         b. F
         c. T
         d. F
         e. F

An accurate estimate of a natural history of rheumatoid arthritis is difficult to obtain since it is difficult to identify and follow-up all cases occurring in the community. A recent review of the long-term prognosis of rheumatoid arthritis was criticised on the grounds of undue selection bias of the more severe cases by a specialist centre (Scott DL *et al.* (1986) Br J Rheumatol 25 Abstr. Suppl. 1 No. 6).

2. Immunology and Infectious Arthritis

Q.2.1 **These statements are true of human immunoglobulins:**

    a. Composed of two heavy chains and two light chains
    b. Heavy chains and light chains are linked by disulphide linkage
    c. Light chains are either kappa or lambda
    d. The heavy chain portion confers specificity
    e. All of the above

Q.2.2 **Prostaglandins**

    a. are low molecular weight polypeptides
    b. are chemically related to thromboxanes
    c. have been clearly shown to be responsible for destruction of cartilage in man
    d. inhibit the secretion of renin
    e. are produced in the seminal vesicles

Q.2.3 **The ESR**

    a. is abnormal in hereditary spherocytosis
    b. is affected by plasma protein concentration
    c. varies with age
    d. is spuriously lowered in anaemia
    e. is higher in males than females
    f. is elevated in pregnancy

Q.2.4 **The following may be elevated as part of the acute phase response:**

    a. Plasma viscosity
    b. Ferritin
    c. Alkaline phosphatase
    d. Haptoglobin
    e. Fibrinogen

Q.2.5 **The following are cytokines:**

    a. Transferrin
    b. Interleukin I
    c. Tumour necrosis factor
    d. Prostaglandin E2
    e. Gamma Interferon

For answers see over

Answers

A.2.1 a. T
        b. T
        c. T
        d. T
        e. T

A.2.2 a. F—They are unsaturated fatty acids containing a cyclopentane ring.
        b. T
        c. F—Their action is mainly on the vascular endothelium.
        d. F—Prostaglandins of the E series increase renin secretion.
        e. T

A.2.3 a. F—The ESR is not affected by the size of the blood cells.
        b. T—Especially fibrinogen.
        c. T—The upper limit of normal rises with age.
        d. F—The ESR is spuriously elevated in anaemia.
        e. F—Not related to sex.
        f. T

A.2.4 a. T
        b. T
        c. T
        d. T
        e. T

All of these may be elevated as part of the acute phase response; ferritin, alkaline phosphatase, haptoglobin and fibrinogen originating in the liver.

A.2.5 a. F
        b. T
        c. T
        d. F
        e. T

Cytokines are defined as soluble molecules produced by white cells which have an effect on the metabolism and function of other cells involved in the inflammatory process. Prostaglandins are potent vasodilators and enhance other mediators of the inflammatory process.

Q.2.6 **Match the following:**

  a. HLA-B27
  b. HLA-DR2
  c. HLA-DR3
  d. HLA-DR4
  e. C4 null alleles
  f. HLA-B5

  A. Found in 60% of subject with rheumatoid arthritis
  B. Associated with a liability to lupus-like syndromes
  C. Associated with milder disease and better response to second-line treatment in rheumatoid arthritis
  D. Associated with susceptibility to renal side-effects of gold treatment
  E. A high population frequency in Turkey
  F. Found in 7% of Caucasians

Q.2.7 **Damage due to oxygen free radicals may play an important part in the maintenance of joint damage in rheumatoid arthritis. The following statements are true:**

  a. Most oxygen free radicals originate in neutrophils
  b. Hydroxyl is the most damaging
  c. Oxygen free radicals may result as a consequence of reperfusion injury
  d. In chronic granulomatous disease patients are unable to manufacture these radicals
  e. NSAIDs inhibit the production of these radicals

For answers see over

Answers

A.2.6 a. F
  b. C
  c. D
  d. A
  e. B—Hydrallazine-induced lupus is more liable to occur in those who are DR4 positive.
  f. E—B5 is associated with Behçet's syndrome.

A.2.7 a. T
  b. F—Hydrogen peroxide is able to cross cell membranes and is potentially most damaging.
  c. T—This has been shown experimentally and is hypothesised to occur in man. The period of hypoperfusion occurs in the knee during walking when intra-articular pressure exceeds capillary perfusion pressure.
  d. T—And these patients are susceptible to bacterial infection.
  e. F

Q.2.8 Assertion/Reason (see p. vi):

Statement 1   Rheumatoid factor is found in approximately 70% of cases of rheumatoid arthritis

Statement 2   Rheumatoid factor is predominantly IgM and is produced in response to a specific antigenic stimulus

Answer key:

Answer	First statement	Second statement	
a.	T	T	Second statement correctly explains first
b.	T	T	Second statement does *not* explain first
c.	T	F	
d.	F	T	
e.	F	F	

Q.2.9 Systemic amyloidosis

a. occurs in a majority of patients who have had rheumatoid arthritis for more than 10 years
b. commonly presents with proteinuria
c. when complicating rheumatoid arthritis is likely to be fatal within five years
d. may be monitored by measuring serum amyloid A
e. may be successfully treated with colchicine

Q.2.10 Septic arthritis may be life-threatening and may rapidly lead to destruction of the joints. Early diagnosis and treatment are essential. The following measures are appropriate:

a. Open surgical drainage is mandatory
b. Intra-articular antibiotics are recommended initially
c. At least three months' treatment with two antibiotics is necessary
d. It is important to maintain the passive range of movement of the joint
e. Diagnosis depends on isolation of bacteria from the joint

For answers see over

Answers

A.2.8   c.   Rheumatoid factor is not an antibody produced to a specific stimulus and may occur in many situations involving chronic inflammation. Rheumatoid factors are possibly useful in the sense that they may crosslink specific IgG antibodies thus facilitating clearance of antibody/antigen complex. They normally vanish in the absence of stimulation but in rheumatoid arthritis may persist due to a lack of galactosyl transferase during active disease.

A.2.9   a.   F—Estimates vary from 5%–20% for clinically overt amyloid although this proportion may be higher if the presence of amyloid is determined solely on rectal biopsy specimens.
      b.   T
      c.   T
      d.   F—Serum amyloid A is an acute phase protein indistinguishable from amyloid deposits in the tissues. However, there seems to be little relationship between the steady-state serum value of amyloid A and the development of amyloidosis. However, diseases not having much of an acute phase response such as systemic lupus erythematosus rarely cause amyloid. On the other hand, in conditions where the acute phase response frequently occurs such as systemic juvenile chronic arthritis and rheumatoid arthritis, amyloidosis is commonly seen.
      e.   F—Except in Familial Mediterranean Fever.

A.2.10   a.   F—The only indication for surgical drainage now is acute septic arthritis of the hip in childhood. Repeated aspiration of pus is usually sufficient in other cases.
      b.   F—Since intra-articular levels of systemic antibiotics are usually adequate.
      c.   F—Although two antibiotics are initially recommended, only one appropriate antibiotic is necessary for the full course of treatment. Some rheumatologists would be satisfied with 6–8 weeks treatment in total.
      d.   T—Although initially pain may prevent anything but minimal passive movement. A resting splint is also useful.
      e.   T—Together with an appropriate cellular synovial exudate. Neutrophil counts generally exceed 100 000.

Q.2.11 **The following organisms commonly cause septic arthritis:**

    a. *Campylobacter jejuni*
    b. *Staphylococcus aureus*
    c. *Escherichia coli*
    d. *Shigella flexneri*
    e. *Mycobacterium tuberculosis*

Q.2.12 **AIDS produces profound abnormalities of the immune system. The following statements are true:**

    a. Having AIDS decreases the chances of developing an auto-immune disease such as rheumatoid arthritis
    b. Human immunotropic virus (HIV) is a risk factor for atypical seronegative arthritis.
    c. HIV is a cause of sexually acquired reactive arthritis
    d. Patients with AIDS are particularly susceptible to septic arthritis

Q.2.13 **The following statements are true of Lyme disease:**

    a. The causative organism is a spirochaete
    b. Chronic arthritis is found in 30% of cases
    c. There is a characteristic rash
    d. Neurological complications may occur
    e. Forestry workers are susceptible

For answers see over

Answers

A.2.11 a. F
 b. T
 c. T
 d. F
 e. F

Theoretically, septic arthritis can be caused by any organism which causes a septicaemia. Arthritis may well be associated with *Shigella flexneri* but usually as a reactive arthritis. A similar argument applies to *Campylobacter*. The most common organism isolated from septic joints in adults is *Staphylococcus aureus*, and in children *Escherichia coli*. Tuberculosis is still an important but, in this country, rare cause of a chronic monarthritis.

A.2.12 a. Theoretically true, because AIDS causes a selective deficiency of CD4 + helper lymphocytes. No firm evidence on this point is available.
 b. T—2%–3% of sexually acquired HIV positive cases develop an atypical seronegative, presumably reactive, arthritis. Arthritis is not seen in transfusion HIV positive cases, thereby suggesting a simultaneously acquired arthritogenic agent.
 c. T—Although the virus has been isolated from inflamed joints.
 d. T—Patients with AIDS are unable to mount an antibody response. They are susceptible to opportunistic infection, characteristically pneumocystis pneumonia and cryptococcus arthritis.

A.2.13 a. T—The organism is *Borrelia burgdorferi* transmitted by a vector, usually an animal tick (*Ixodes*).
 b. T
 c. T—Typically erythema chronica migrans appears preceding the onset of arthritis and other complications.
 d. T—Including encephalitis, fits and neuropathy.
 e. T—Originally described in Lyme, Massachusetts, where the ticks originated on deer. In the UK cases have been reported from the New Forest.

Q.2.14   The arthritis associated with Rubella

    a. involves small joints more frequently than large joints
    b. may follow Rubella vaccination
    c. is usually a temporary synovitis concurrent with the rash
    d. may result in Rubella virus being obtained from synovial fluid
    e. is associated with characteristic radiological changes in the affected joints

Q.2.15   Match the following:

    a. Clutton's joints
    b. Poncet's arthritis
    c. Jaccoud's arthropathy
    d. Reiter's syndrome
    e. Lyme arthritis

    A. *Shigella flexneri*
    B. *Mycobacterium tuberculosis*
    C. *Treponema pallidum*
    D. Group A haemolytic *Streptococcus*
    E. *Borrelia burgdorferi*

Q.2.16   In rheumatoid arthritis, septic arthritis is a common complication. The following statements are true:

    a. In subjects on steroids the usual signs of infection may be obscured.
    b. Infection rarely occurs in more than one joint at a time
    c. The commonest infecting organism is *Staphylococcus aureus*
    d. Antibiotic treatment should be administered intra-articularly
    e. Surgical drainage is mandatory

For answers see over

Answers

A.2.14 a. F—Usually larger joints.
      b. T—In 15% of cases.
      c. F—The arthritis, usually a temporary synovitis, occurs after the rash has appeared.
      d. T
      e. F—Usually this is a non-erosive, non-deforming, self-limiting arthritis.

A.2.15 a. C
      b. B
      c. D
      d. A
      e. E

A.2.16 a. T.
      b. F—Multiple septic joints do occur and this condition may occur without systemic signs of infection but with such features as general deterioration in mobility, weight loss, and increased pain in the joints. If in doubt, aspirate.
      c. T—In 90% of cases the organism is *Staphylococcus aureus*.
      d. F—Adequate intra-articular levels of antibiotics are achieved with intravenous or oral therapy. The duration of treatment is important: two to three months is recommended.
      e. F—A similar outcome has been shown in matched surgically and conservatively treated joints. In childhood this may not be the case and surgical drainage is recommended, especially in cases of hip infection.

3. Clinical Pharmacology

Q.3.1 **Slow acetylators are more prone to the following adverse drug effects:**

a. Haemolysis with methyldopa
b. Hepatitis with isoniazid
c. Nausea and vomiting with sulphasalazine
d. Peripheral neuropathy with isoniazid
e. Systemic lupus syndrome with hydrallazine

Q.3.2 **It is known that non-steroidal anti-inflammatory drugs frequently produce side-effects. The following statements are true:**

a. Non-steroidal anti-inflammatory drugs are probably the drugs of choice for treating acute gout
b. These drugs are more likely to cause gastrointestinal disturbance in the elderly
c. They should never be given as long courses
d. Where gastric intolerance is a problem, non-steroidal anti-inflammatory drugs may be used as suppositories
e. Men on non-steroidal anti-inflammatory drugs are more prone to peptic ulcer complications than women

Q.3.3 **Local steroid injections are a useful treatment in**

a. ganglion
b. Achilles paratendinitis
c. ischial bursitis
d. de Quervain's tenosynovitis
e. carpal tunnel syndrome

For answers see over

Answers

A.3.1 a. F
        b. F—This is more common in fast acetylators.
        c. T
        d. T
        e. T
Side-effects with isoniazid, sulphasalazine (and its metabolites) and hydrallazine are dose-dependant and therefore more often seen in slow acetylators.

A.3.2 a. T—Any will do but indomethacin, up to 200 mg daily, is very effective.
        b. T—The elderly are more prone to perforation and bleeding.
        c. F—In chronic inflammatory states such as rheumatoid arthritis, regular long-term dosage is often necessary.
        d. T—Although the problems are not eliminated. Concurrent use of H2 blockers may also help.
        e. F—No sex difference.

A.3.3 a. T
        b. T—Although some orthopaedic surgeons would shy away from injecting Achilles paratendinitis because of the risk of subsequent rupture. This risk seems slight if a soluble preparation such as hydrocortisone is used and the injection is placed around and not in the tendon itself.
        c. T
        d. T
        e. T

Q.3.4 **The following drugs have been demonstrated to alter the progression of rheumatoid arthritis as assessed by X-ray examination:**

a. Aspirin
b. Gold
c. Methotrexate
d. Penicillamine
e. Corticosteroids

Q.3.5 **When treating elderly patients with arthritis**

a. once-daily medication is preferable for the patient
b. paracetamol is a good anti-inflammatory agent
c. acute exacerbations may be due to septic arthritis
d. steroids have no place in treatment
e. non-steroidal anti-inflammatory drugs and anti-depressants should not be given together

For answers see over

Answers

A.3.4 a. F

b. T—The Empire Rheumatism Council trial of gold in the late 1950s demonstrated less progression of erosions in the treated as opposed to the control group.

c. F

d. F

e. T—The MRC and Nuffield Foundation steroid trial in 1959 demonstrated the ability of low dose steroid to retard the progression of erosions.

Whereas "disease-modifying" anti-rheumatic drugs have an effect on the clinical and laboratory indices of inflammation, evidence that these drugs retard radiological progression is surprisingly sparse and extremely difficult to obtain. This is in part due to the logistic and ethical difficulties in establishing appropriate placebo controls for a period of time long enough to demonstrate radiological changes. This was less of a problem in the late 1950s.

A.3.5 a. T—A once-daily regime aids compliance, although caution is advised lest accumulation of the drug occurs.

b. F—Paracetamol is an analgesic with no anti-inflammatory effect. However, its analgesic properties may be sufficient to relieve symptoms.

c. T—A septic arthritis is not uncommon in the elderly and the classical signs of infection may not always be present. In a sick elderly patient with arthritis, always suspect a septic joint and aspirate any suspicious joints.

d. F—Corticosteroids may be effective in relieving acute flares of rheumatoid arthritis and occasionally for maintenance.

e: F—Associated depression may be the cause of a poor response to anti-inflammatory treatment.

Q.3.6 **The effects of corticosteroids on inflammation include**

    a. stabilisation of lysosomal membrane
    b. reversal of enhanced capillary permeability
    c. increased exudation of inflammatory cells from vascular tree
    d. increase in circulating neutrophil count
    e. none of the above

Q.3.7 **The figure represents the single oral dose pharmacokinetic profile of a non-steroidal anti-inflammatory drug. The following statements are true:**

    a. The $t_{\frac{1}{2}}$ of this drug is six hours
    b. The drug need only be administered once daily
    c. Significant accumulation of the drug may occur when given once daily in elderly subjects
    d. The best indicator of drug efficacy is its peak plasma concentration
    e. The pharmacokinetic profile is independent of the time of administration of the drug
    f. The pharmacokinetic profile is unlikely to change if the drug is administered with milk

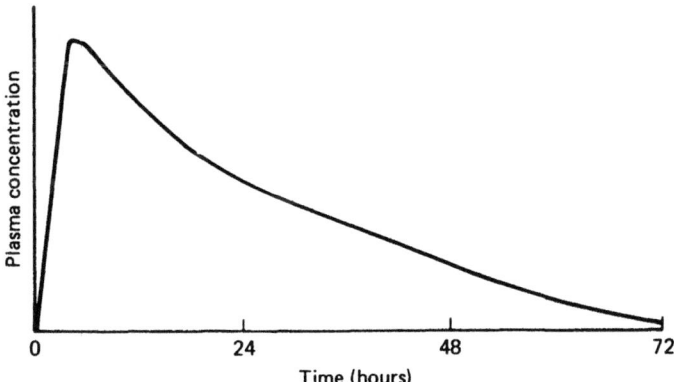

For answers see over

Answers

A.3.6 a. T
       b. T
       c. F—There is a reduction in extravascular exudation of inflammatory cells.
       d. T
       e. F

Steroids exert their anti-inflammatory effect in a number of ways including antagonism of the kallikrein-kinin system and inhibition of prostaglandin release from stimulated cells. They have a noticeable effect on the peripheral lymphocyte count causing a decrease in circulating T lymphocytes.

A.3.7 a. F—The $t_{\frac{1}{2}}$ is 24 hours and is the time to reach half the maximum plasma concentration.
       b. T
       c. T—Usually separate studies in the elderly are required for product licences. This is especially so with non-steroidal anti-inflammatory drugs where impaired renal function may cause accumulation and where non-steroidal anti-inflammatory drug therapy may cause a decrease in renal function by their effect on renal blood flow.
       d. F—The best indicator of a drug's efficacy is a clinical response. The pharmacokinetic variable most likely to correlate with this is the intra-synovial concentration.
       e. F—Studies have shown different pharmacokinetic profiles when the drug is given at different times of day.
       f. F—Some non-steroidal anti-inflammatory drugs are lipid soluble, for example nabumetone, and show higher plasma levels when given with lipid-containing fluids such as milk.

Q.3.8 **The following scenario would alert you to potential drug interactions:**

a. A 70-year-old male being treated for hypertension and congestive cardiac failure is started on piroxicam for osteoarthritis of the hip

b. A 40-year-old female taking methotrexate for her psoriasis is started on mefenamic acid for low back pain

c. A 60-year-old male on theophylline for his chest and ibuprofen for his osteoarthritic knees is given cimetidine for his dyspepsia

d. An 80-year-old female on benorylate for chronic rheumatoid arthritis requests additional analgesia. Paracetamol up to 4 g daily in divided doses is given

e. A 45-year-old male with a history of typical podagra is given allopurinol and indomethacin concurrently

Q.3.9 **The following are potential side-effects of non-steroidal anti-inflammatory agents:**

a. Headache

b. Confusion

c. Interstitial nephritis

d. Elevated serum creatinine

e. Oedema

For answers see over

Answers

A.3.8 a–d contain possible therapeutic mishaps.

a. Piroxicam may antagonise the antihypertensive effect of such drugs as beta blockers and ACE inhibitors. Furthermore, non-steroidal anti-inflammatory drugs may cause fluid and water retention thus producing a deterioration in congestive cardiac failure.

b. Non-steroidal anti-inflammatory drugs such as mefenamic acid may potentiate methotrexate by reduction of renal tubular excretion and displacement from binding sites.

c. Cimetidine as an inhibitor of drug metabolising enzymes in the liver may potentiate the effect of drugs mainly cleared by hepatic metabolism such as theophyllines.

d. Benorylate is metabolised after absorption to salicylate and paracetamol. On a standard dose of 4-g benorylate twice daily almost 4-g paracetamol are obtained (and 4.5-g aspirin). Therefore, additional paracetamol may exceed the ability of the liver to metabolise this drug, leading to paracetamol toxicity.

e. When starting allopurinol as a prophylactic treatment for gout, a non-steroidal anti-inflammatory drug should be given concurrently for the first three months to help prevent the acute episodes of gout which are occasionally precipitated.

A.3.9 a. T
b. T
c. T
d. T
e. T

The elevated serum creatinine and decreased creatinine clearance together with oedema are probably due to antagonism of prostaglandin mediated changes in renal blood flow.

Q.3.10A   A 50-year-old white female is referred to out-patients . She has a 3-year history of early morning stiffness and intermittent pain in the knees and hands. On examination she has symmetrical soft tissue swelling of the mcp joints of both hands, subcutaneous nodules and mild flexion deformities of her knees. The GP has treated her with gold 50 mg intramuscularly weekly for the last three months with some benefit but the patient has recently developed severe diarrhoea. She has also been taking aspirin 0.9 g q.d.s. with benefit but considerable indigestion. You should

a. continue gold to a total dose of 1g and then review
b. stop gold immediately and start steroids
c. stop gold and aspirin immediately and start another non-steroidal anti-inflammatory drug
d. refer the patient to the physiotherapy department

Q.3.10B   Investigation of the above patient reveals an ESR of 80, an SCAT of 1 in 256, an ANF 1 in 1000, erosions of both hands and feet, and a small pleural effusion on chest X-ray films. You should

a. change the diagnosis to SLE and start steroids immediately
b. look for an alternative cause for the pulmonary effusion
c. start on alternative second-line therapy, for example D-penicillamine, after checking blood and urine and after the bowels have settled
d. ask the laboratory for further tests of antinuclear factor to define exactly the nature of this antibody

For answers see over

Answers

A.3.10A   a. F
              b. F
              c. T
              d. T

Gold may cause a severe haemorrhagic colitis and the drug should be discontinued at the first suggestion of this complication. There is no indication for steroids in this case at the present and the diarrhoea should resolve on cessation of gold treatment. If haemorrhagic colitis develops then appropriate fluid and electrolyte replacement must be started together with systemic steroids. The patient should be referred to the physiotherapy department for education on her disease and instruction on how to overcome flexion deformity of her knees and in order to prevent any deformity occurring in the hands.

A.3.10B   a. F
              b. T
              c. F
              d. T

15% of patients with rheumatoid arthritis have a positive antinuclear factor. This titre is however rather high and it may be worth seeking confirmation of a co-existing diagnosis of SLE by asking for further definition of the antibodies. Pleural effusion may be compatible with SLE and a search must be made for possible renal disease. Skin biopsy may be helpful where, even in a normal area of skin, characteristic immunohistological features may be found.

It must never be assumed that co-existing pleural effusion is due to the rheumatoid disease and appropriate diagnostic aspiration must be undertaken together with any other pulmonary investigations indicated. A rheumatoid pleural effusion characteristically is sterile with a high protein and low glucose and may often be rheumatoid factor positive.

D-penicillamine is best avoided even if rheumatoid arthritis is thought to be the diagnosis, because this drug may, on occasion, induce SLE.

Q.3.10C DNA binding is normal and nucleolar protein antibodies are negative. Sulphasalazine is started and increased steadily to a dose of 2 g daily. After 6 months the patient is clinically improved, the ESR has fallen and the pleural effusion resolved. You should now

    a. stop sulphasalazine

    b. increase sulphasalazine to 3 g daily to obtain maximum benefit

    c. continue sulphasalazine in this dose and check blood and urine weekly for side-effects

    d. none of the above

Q.3.11 The following may be a toxic manifestation of gold:

    a. Haemorrhagic colitis

    b. Elevated transaminases

    c. Haematuria

    d. Leucopenia

    e. Thrombocytopenia

    f. All of the above

Does oral gold have a similar spectrum of side-effects?

Q.3.12 The following is the least common manifestation of aspirin ingestion:

    a. Duodenal ulcer

    b. Haemorrhagic gastritis

    c. Positive faecal occult blood

    d. Low serum iron

    e. Low ferritin

For answers see over

Answers

A.3.10C a. F
             b. F
             c. F
             d. T

If sulphasalazine is effective at 2 g daily it should be continued at this dose with monthly blood checks for thrombocytopenia or leucopenia. If, after a period, the effect of the sulphasalazine appears to wear off then the dose may be further increased to 3 g in order to obtain additional benefit, but it must be recognised that side-effects from this drug are probably dose-related.

A.3.11 a. T
          b. T
          c. T
          d. T
          e. T
          f. T

Oral gold (Auranofin) has a similar side-effect profile though side-effects are less severe and similar precautions should be taken during its administration. Diarrhoea is the most frequent side-effect or oral gold; the stool frequency may be controlled by temporary reduction in dosage. Rarely, as with intramuscular gold, a haemorrhagic enterocolitis may develop.

A.3.12 a. T
          b. F
          c. F
          d. F
          e. F

Tests for faecal occult blood are frequently positive in patients on aspirin and radiolabelled red blood cell studies show an increase in the daily loss of blood from the gastrointestinal tract due to subclinical gastritis. Ultimately this may lead to a low serum iron and iron deficiency anaemia.

Q.3.13 **The following statements are true of analgesics:**

a. The analgesic effect of aspirin increases up to but not exceeding 1 g four times a day
b. Paracetamol has major analgesic and anti-inflammatory actions
c. Paracetamol does not usually produce gastrointestinal bleeding or dyspepsia
d. Diarrhoea is a side-effect of codeine phosphate
e. Ibuprofen is analgesic up to 600 mg daily and thereafter has analgesic and anti-inflammatory action

Q.3.14 **A patient with arthritis on non-steroidal anti-inflammatory drugs (NSAIDs) complains of dyspepsia. You should**

a. review the diagnosis and consider using a pure analgesic instead
b. stop the drug pending gastrointestinal investigation
c. give the non-steroidal anti-inflammatory drug as a suppository in order to reduce the risk of gastrointestinal symptoms and ulcer
d. give a H_2-blocker in order to reduce the risk of gastrointestinal symptoms and ulcer
e. give a prostaglandin analogue, now generally available, which protects against corrosive damage of the upper gastrointestinal tract produced by non-steroidal anti-inflammatory drugs

Q.3.15 **Match the following:**

a. Causes a reduction in synovial interleukin 1 levels
b. Induces a reduction in circulating B lymphocytes
c. A sulphonamide moiety provides the anti-rheumatic activity
d. Causes an increase in circulating B lymphocytes
e. Alleviates morning stiffness

A. Ibuprofen
B. Sulphasalazine
C. Nefopam
D. Sodium aurothiomalate
E. Steroids

For answers see over

Answers

A.3.13
a. T—Aspirin has analgesic, antipyretic and anti-inflammatory properties. As an analgesic the usual dose is up to 600 mg four times a day.

b. F—Paracetamol is as effective as aspirin in relieving pain but has no anti-inflammatory action.

c. T

d. F—Codeine and di-hydrocodeine are useful analgesics but may produce dizziness and constipation as side-effects.

e. T—The analgesic action of ibuprofen and other non-steroidal anti-inflammatory drugs is mediated peripherally.

A.3.14
a. T—If the diagnosis is osteoarthrosis without any obvious inflammatory component, it is always worth persisting with analgesics in the first instance since these and physiotherapy may be readily effective in relieving pain and improving function.

b. F—Non-ulcer dyspepsia may occur with non-steroidal anti-inflammatory drugs but it is worth reducing the dose.

c. T—Giving the drug as a suppository does not eliminate this risk, though it may reduce it.

d. T—Even proven ulcers have been shown to heal while patients continue with NSAID therapy and take concomitant H_2-blockers.

e. T.

A.3.15
a. A
b. D
c. B
d. E
e. C

Q.3.16 **Local steroid injections are a vital therapeutic option in rheumatology. The following statement applies:**

a. The duration of action of the injection is dependent on the solubility of the preparation used

b. Microcrystalline preparations of steroid may themselves cause a brief exacerbation of joint symptoms

c. Intra-articular injections into weight-bearing joints should be followed by a 1-week period of complete bed-rest

d. Repeated intra-articular steroids may cause a Charcot-like arthropathy

e. Injection of steroid into tendon sheaths is not recommended

Q.3.17 **Before a drug claiming to have disease-modifying activity in rheumatoid arthritis can be licensed in the UK, the following data are needed:**

a. The marketing company must have at least 10 years' experience with the drug in patients with rheumatoid arthritis

b. Absence of teratogenicity in animals on exposure to therapeutic concentrations of the drug

c. Favourable radiological evidence over a 12-month period in comparison with placebo in patients with active rheumatoid arthritis

d. Disease remission must have occurred in at least 50% of trial patients within six months

e. None of the above

For answers see over

Answers

A.3.16 a. T—Ranging from the soluble suspension of hydrocortisone to the longer acting crystalline preparations of methylprednisolone and triamcinolone.

        b. T—Occurring within 24 h of injection; some estimates are as high as 15%.

        c. F—Whereas this may have been the practice some years ago, nowadays 24–48 h bed-rest is recommended for full therapeutic effect. When using the longer acting preparations, it is important to warn the patient that the full benefit may not be evident for 1–2 weeks.

        d. T—Although this risk has been over-estimated and is based on cases having frequent (weekly) injections over a prolonged period.

        e. F—Although the more soluble preparations should be used.

A.3.17 a. F
        b. F
        c. F
        d. F
        e. T

A new drug must have data relating to toxicology in animals but a teratogenic drug is not excluded (although if present, women with child-bearing potential are likely to be excluded). The manufacturer must show it to have an acceptable therapeutic ratio. It must be shown to be free from serious side-effects in normal volunteers and patients, including the elderly. Pharmacokinetic and safety data are also needed for a group of patients similar to those for whom the drug is intended.

Q.3.18 **The following statements are true about gold treatment:**

  a. A standard course of chrysotherapy involves weekly intramuscular injections of 50 mg gold up to a total dose of 1 g, or until clinical improvement occurs, following which treatment should be discontinued

  b. Following treatment with gold, the drug may reside in the tissues for up to one year

  c. ·Proteinuria is the commonest reason for withdrawing the drug

  d. Renal toxicity is more likely if the patient has previously developed proteinuria on D-penicillamine

  e. If the patient responds to gold and then subsequently relapses on maintenance treatment, an increased dose may induce further remission

Q.3.19 **A 42-year-old male with rheumatoid arthritis is started on gold. Three months later this treatment is stopped because of significant proteinuria. Sulphasalazine is started. Three months later thrombocytopenia is found. These changes are indicated in the figure. The following statements are true:**

  a. A bone marrow examination is unlikely to be helpful

  b. The thrombocytopenia may be due to gold

  c. Thrombocytopenia due to sulphasalazine occurs in about 1% of those treated

  d. Sulphasalazine should be stopped and oral steroids started

  e. Penicillamine is contraindicated in this patient

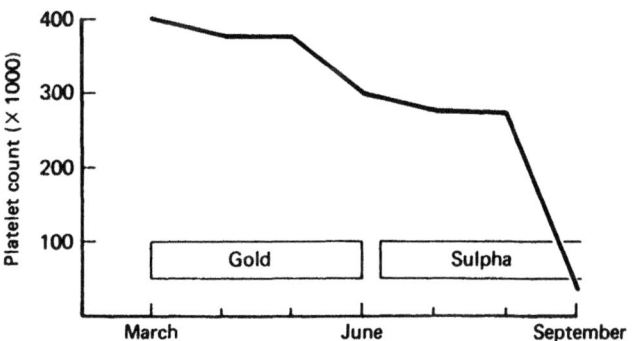

For answers see over

Answers

A.3.18 a. F—If clinical improvement occurs after the initial course then the frequency of the injections should always be reduced rather than the drug discontinued.

b. T .

c. F—Rash is the commonest reason and occurs in up to 30% of people started on gold.

d. T—But this does not mean gold is contra-indicated in these circumstances.

e. T

A.3.19 a. T—The mechanism of gold-induced thrombocytopenia is not clear but marrow examination usually reveals normal numbers of megakaryocytes.

b. T—Side-effects such as these may occur following cessation of gold therapy for up to 6 months.

c. F—Neutropenia is the commonest haematological complication following sulphasalazine therapy and occurs in just under 5% of those treated. Thrombocytopenia is a rare complication.

d. T—In view of the platelet count.

e. F—Although it is recommended that a 6-month period following cessation of gold or sulphasalazine therapy be observed to minimise subsequent side-effects with penicillamine.

4. Juvenile Arthritis

Q.4.1 **In juvenile chronic arthritis**

   a. rheumatoid factor, identical to that occurring in adult disease, is found in the majority of cases

   b. those patients with polyarticular disease are at risk from blindness due to insidiously progressive iridocyclitis

   c. in the majority, the functional outlook beyond the age of 20 years is good

   d. all classes of disease are at risk from systemic amyloidosis

   e. about 1 in 6 have a B27 associated spondarthropathy

Q.4.2 **In systemic onset juvenile chronic arthritis (Still's disease)**

   a. the majority have a positive sheep cell agglutination test

   b. aortic incompetence is a recognised complication

   c. the prognosis as regards disability is better than with adult rheumatoid arthritis

   d. the cervical spine is often involved

   e. cataract may occur

Q.4.3 **In Henoch–Schönlein purpura**

   a. the knee joints are most frequently involved

   b. the rash rarely occurs on the arms

   c. abdominal colic may occur

   d. incidence peaks in pre-school children

   e. haematuria may occur

Q.4.4 **In the differential diagnosis of a limp in a child**

   a. pain is not a typical feature of Perthes' disease of the hip

   b. hip pain may follow an upper respiratory tract infection

   c. the limp often precedes pain in slipped upper femoral epiphysis

   d. Osgood–Schlatter's disease may be the cause

   e. osteochondritis dissecans may be the cause

For answers see over

Answers

A.4.1 a. F—Rheumatoid factor is present in the minority, about 12%, and usually in those with juvenile rheumatoid-type arthritis.

       b. F—Usually the pauciarticular types (less than four joints) are at risk, especially if anti-nuclear factor positive. This group must be checked regularly by an ophthalmologist even if asymptomatic.

       c. T

       d. F—Only those with systemic onset classical Still's disease are at risk of amyloidosis. A genetic marker has now been identified. The quoted frequency of this complication is 10% in 10 years.

       e. T

A.4.2 a. F—Fewer than 50% are positive for rheumatoid factor.

       b. F—Serositis and especially pericarditis may occur but endocarditis is rarely seen.

       c. T—Although deformity at adolescence may be marked, many of these patients cope well with their disability in adult life.

       d. T—Causing cervical fusion.

       e. T—This complication is more frequently seen in patients with pauci-articular arthritis with positive antinuclear antibodies.

A.4.3 a. T

       b. T

       c. T

       d. T

       e. T

Knees, ankles, hip, elbows and wrists may be involved but there is a preponderance of lower limb involvement. Affected joints may show effusions with a high white cell count, mainly of polymorphs. Complete resolution is the rule.

A.4.4 a. F—In the majority of cases of Perthes' disease pain is present at the onset. About a quarter are painless initially.

       b. T—Causing the so-called transient post-streptococcal synovitis.

       c. T—This is occasionally bilateral (in about a quarter).

       d. F—Osgood–Schlatter's disease or tibial epiphysitis may cause pain over the tibial tubercle in older children but does not usually cause a limp.

       e. T

Q.4.5 Acute systemic onset juvenile chronic arthritis (Still's disease) and Kawasaki's disease may easily be confused. The following features would favour the diagnosis of Kawasaki's disease:

a. A high swinging fever
b. Lymphadenopathy
c. Peeling of skin on the fingers
d. Polyarthritis
e. Good response to steroids

Q.4.6 In children, acute leukaemia may present with

a. generalised arthralgia
b. irritable hip
c. hydrarthrosis
d. a positive rheumatoid factor
e. generalised myalgia

Q.4.7 These features are characteristic of systemic onset juvenile chronic arthritis (Still's disease):

a. Fever
b. Rash
c. Latex positivity
d. Splenomegaly
e. Lymphadenopathy
f. All of the above

For answers see over

Answers

A.4.5 a. F
b. F
c. T
d. F
e. F

These syndromes may easily be confused. One distinguishing feature is peeling skin on the hands and feet in Kawasaki's disease. Because there is involvement of the coronary sinus and coronary arteries, and some people feel this may be exacerbated by steroids, steroids are contra-indicated in this disease.

A.4.6 a. T
b. T—Possibly due to infiltration of capsule and periosteum.
c. T
d. F
e. T

Other clinical features to suggest a diagnosis of leukaemia are an ill child with fever, purpura, lymphadenopathy and hepatosplenomegaly. Lymph node biopsy may be misleading since the pathological features of rheumatoid arthritis may mimic those of a lymphoma.

A.4.7 a. T
b. T
c. F
d. T
e. T
f. F

The rash usually consists of discrete pink macules on the trunk, face and extremities. Usually the rash is only present for a short period of time coincidental with the spikes of fever. The fever is said to be characteristic, with extremely wide variation in temperature over the course of a day with, usually, one high spike towards the late evening. The fever may precede the onset of arthritis by many weeks. The latex test is rarely positive, probably in 10%–20% at diagnosis.

Q.4.8 **You often meet sacroiliitis, micrognathia, arthritis of the apophyseal joints of the cervical spine, and occasional anky-losis of the affected joints in the following conditions:**

a. Rheumatoid arthritis
b. Reiter's syndrome
c. Juvenile chronic arthritis
d. Rheumatic fever
e. Infectious arthritis

Q.4.9 **The management of juvenile chronic arthritis requires expertise from several different specialities. The following statements apply specifically to juvenile chronic arthritis:**

a. Splinting of inflamed joints is not recommended because it leads to joint contractures
b. Arthritis may lead to premature fusion of the epiphyses and consequent shortening of a limb
c. Arthritis may cause overgrowth necessitating surgical intervention
d. A patient may apply for a mobility allowance regardless of youth
e. As adults, these patients do not have any particular anaesthetic problems

Q.4.10 **In the treatment of juvenile chronic arthritis**

a. corticosteroids have little suppressive effect on the hypothalamo-pituitary axis provided they are given in a dose not greater than 2.0 mg/kg on alternate days
b. if growth retardation is severe, an increase in growth may be seen after starting steroid treatment
c. aspirin is still the best first choice non-steroidal anti-inflammatory drug
d. conventional disease-modifying agents are of proven benefit in all classes of disease
e. cytotoxic therapy may be required

For answers see over

Answers

A.4.8 a. F
b. F
c. T
d. F
e. F

A.4.9 a. F—Rest splints are used to try to prevent the formation of contractures.
b. T—This is most dramatically seen with micrognathia.
c. T—If the medial femoral condyle and adjacent tibial plateau are affected, then a resulting valgus deformity of the knee may occur.
d. T—Only the elderly, i.e., those over 65 years of age when first applying, cannot obtain a mobility allowance.
e. F—Anaesthetic problems are particularly apparent in later life with such deformities as micrognathia and cervical spine fusion.

A.4.10 a. T
b. T—Although caution must be used in the application of this advice since steroids themselves may suppress growth in children. If the systemic features of the disease are severe enough to cause growth retardation, then treatment with systemic corticosteroids may produce an acceleration in growth rate.
c. F—Aspirin is now not recommended for children due to the association of aspirin with Reye's syndrome. In addition, aspirin has a narrow therapeutic dose range.
d. F—Experience with these drugs is limited to use in juvenile rheumatoid arthritis and polyarticular disease only. There is little evidence of efficacy in either except perhaps for gold.
e. T—Especially with systemic amyloidosis where chlorambucil may be indicated.

5. *Seronegative Arthritis*

Q.5.1 **The following conditions are included in the seronegative spondarthritis group of arthritides:**

a. Gout
b. Diffuse idiopathic skeletal hyperostosis
c. Reiter's disease
d. Generalised osteoarthritis
e. Psoriatic arthritis

Q.5.2 **The following clinical features are shared by diseases included in the seronegative spondarthritis group:**

a. Mucocutaneous ulceration
b. Ocular inflammation
c. Psoriasiform skin lesions
d. Familial aggregation
e. Erythema nodosum

Q.5.3 **Assertion/Reason (see p.vi):**

Statement 1   HLA-B27 is found in 50% of subjects with ankylosing spondylitis
Statement 2   *Klebsiella pneumonia* share epitopes with HLA-B27 cell surface markers

Answer key:

Answer	First Statement	Second Statement	
a.	T	T	Second statement correctly explains first
b.	T	T	Second statement does *not* explain first
c.	T	F	
d.	F	T	
e.	F	F	

For answers see over

Answers

A.5.1 a. F
        b. F
        c. T
        d. F
        e. T

The hallmark of diseases in this group of arthritides is bilateral sacroiliitis and a seronegative anodular inflammatory peripheral arthritis. Although diffuse idiopathic skeletal hyperostosis is associated with bony ankylosis of the paravertebral ligaments, sacroiliitis is rarely seen in this condition. Similarly with osteoarthritis, although there is a seronegative anodular occasionally inflammatory peripheral arthritis together with a frequently found degenerative spondylitis, bilateral inflammatory sacroiliitis is not found.

A.5.2 a. T
        b. T
        c. T
        d. T
        e. T

Each condition within this group tends to have a particular feature emphasised, such as skin lesions in psoriatic arthritis, mucocutaneous ulceration in Behçet's disease. However, each disease within this group may exhibit one of the features noted and in addition thrombophlebitis may be found and the diseases share radiological sacroiliitis, ankylosing spondylitis and seronegative peripheral arthritis.

A.5.3 e. HLA-B27 is found in over 90% of subjects with AS. 20% of people carrying the HLA-B27 antigen will develop ankylosing spondylitis at some point. *Klebsiella pneumonia* has been isolated preferentially from subjects with ankylosing spondylitis and some have claimed that *Klebsiella* growth in the stools correlates with disease activity. Serum from patients with ankylosing spondylitis who are B27-positive cross-reacts with *Klebsiella pneumonia* antigens but this work has only been successfully carried out in one centre and the antigenic determinants have not yet been defined.

Q.5.4 **Recognised features of Reiter's syndrome include**

a. balanitis xerotica obliterans
b. calcaneal spurs
c. posterior uveitis
d. sacroiliitis
e. subungual keratosis

Q.5.5 **Ankylosing spondylitis may present with**

a. subcutaneous nodules
b. iritis
c. conjunctivitis
d. inflamed bursae
e. decreased chest expansion
f. peripheral joint involvement

Q.5.6 **Behcet's disease was originally described in Turkey. This disease is now most commonly reported from Japan and the Mediterranean littoral. These statements about Behçet's disease are true:**

a. In Japan it is one of the commonest causes of blindness in young males
b. Japanese emigrating to the USA carry the same risk as indigenous Japanese
c. Major vessel inflammation may lead to strokes and limb gangrene
d. Neurological complications are inevitable
e. Gastrointestinal inflammation leading to pain and melaena may occur

For answers see over

Answers

A.5.4   a. F—Well circumscribed painless superficial red erosions on the glans penis are characteristic; this is also known as circinate balanitis.

        b. T

        c. F—Iritis may occur and conjunctivitis and, occasionally, superficial keratitis but not posterior uveitis.

        d. T

        e. T—This is part of keratoderma blenorrhagica.

A.5.5   a. F—Subcutaneous nodules are more characteristic of rheumatoid arthritis.

        b. T—Some people regard iritis as a separate disease entity existing within the spectrum of seronegative arthritis.

        c. F—This is seen more frequently in Reiter's syndrome.

        d. F—These are more typical of gout and rheumatoid arthritis.

        e. T—This is one of the diagnostic criteria for ankylosing spondylitis.

        f. T—Oligoarthritis, especially of the large joints such as the knee and ankle, may be a presenting feature for many years before back symptoms and signs become evident.

A.5.6   a. T

        b. F—The risk appears to diminish after emigration, thus suggesting some environmental factor is operative in Japan. Speculation has centred on pesticides and organophosphates as well as lead.

        c. T—Both arterial and venous problems may occur.

        d. F—Different sub-groups of Behçet's disease are now recognised. Females with orogenital ulceration appear to follow a benign course without the ocular or neurological complications of this disease.

        e. T

Q.5.7 A 50-year-old male presents with multiple painful ulcers on the tongue and a 2-week history of polyarthritis. Other clinical findings might include

a. circinate balanitis
b. primary chancre
c. posterior choroidoretinitis
d. iritis
e. conjunctivitis

Q.5.8 A 25-year-old female cross-country runner presents with a history of low back pain. The pain is usually worse after particularly arduous events and prevents her from training for several days. Further questioning reveals a history of episodic bloody diarrhoea. On examination no abnormal musculoskeletal signs are present but sigmoidoscopy reveals proctocolitis. An X-ray examination of her back reveals bilateral sacroiliitis. You should

a. perform HLA typing
b. arrange a barium enema to outline the extent of colonic inflammation
c. advise her to stop running
d. prescribe a non-steroidal anti-inflammatory drug
e. warn her about the risk of pregnancy

For answers see over

Answers

A.5.7 a. T
b. T
c. T
d. T
e. T

Circinate balanitis and conjunctivitis may be associated symptoms of Reiter's syndrome. If Reiter's disease is confirmed there may be a co-existing venereal disease. The clinical findings are also compatible with Behçet's disease in which iritis and posterior choroidoretinitis may be found.

A.5.8 a. F—In this sort of case it provides no extra diagnostic or therapeutic information.
b. T—Although her main symptom is low back pain clearly she has bowel inflammation which may be more extensive than the history suggests.
c. F—If, as seems likely, she has spondylitis associated with inflammatory bowel disease then she needs to keep on exercising. In particular, she should be instructed on specific spinal flexibility movements in addition to her general fitness.
d. T—This will help her to train and do her exercises. She should be recommended to take these drugs only on a p.r.n. basis at first. It should also be noted that these drugs may cause a deterioration in her colonic symptoms.
e. F—From the viewpoint of spondylitis, pregnancy sometimes has a beneficial effect on the disease although occasionally it worsens during pregnancy. If she were HLA-B27 positive it could be argued that she should have genetic counselling but since only one-fifth of patients with this antigen develop spinal disease they are often happy to take the risk.

Q.5.9 **Regional enteritis (Crohn's disease) and ulcerative colitis are associated with an arthropathy. The following statements are true about both of these disorders:**

a. The peripheral arthritis often resolves when the disease is successfully treated surgically
b. The arthritis is asymmetrical, non-erosive and seldom destructive
c. The spondylitis responds to treatment of the bowel inflammation with sulphasalazine
d. Iritis may occur
e. Treatment of the peripheral arthritis with non-steroidal anti-inflammatory drugs is contra-indicated

Q.5.10 **The following patterns of arthritis may be associated with psoriasis:**

a. Symmetrical polyarthritis
b. A predominant involvement of distal interphalangeal joints
c. Mutilating arthritis of the hands
d. Asymmetrical oligoarthritis
e. Ankylosing spondylitis

For answers see over

Answers

A.5.9   a. F—This statement is true for ulcerative colitis but not true for Crohn's disease, possibly due to recurrence of inflammation in remaining bowel.
   b. T
   c. F—The spondylitis in both cases appears to progress independently of the bowel inflammation and in some cases has been reported to precede the bowel disease.
   d. T
   e. F—However, caution must be used because of the known side-effects of non-steroidal anti-inflammatory drugs on the gut. These include upper gastro-intestinal ulceration. There have been recent reports of small bowel inflammation due to non-steroidal anti-inflammatory drugs.

A.5.10   a. T—15%
   b. T—5%
   c. T—5%
   d. T—70%
   e. T—5%

Some authors still refuse to believe that psoriatic arthritis exists. They suggest that most of the disease subsets are other forms of arthritis co-existing with psoriasis and that psoriasis may amplify the response to these other arthritides.

Q.5.11 In the treatment of psoriatic arthritis

   a. gold, hydroxychloroquine and sulphasalazine may all be useful
   b. anti-malarial drugs may cause a deterioration in the psoriasis
   c. the severity of the arthritis is directly related to the severity of the psoriasis
   d. methotrexate is useful in the treatment of both the arthritis and the psoriasis
   e. intra-articular steroids are contra-indicated

Q.5.12 The following radiological features may be found in psoriatic arthritis:

   a. Marginal erosions
   b. Syndesmophyte formation
   c. Periostitis
   d. Acro-osteolysis
   e. Erosion of odontoid peg

For answers see over

Answers

A.5.11 a. T—So-called disease-modifying drugs used in rheumatoid arthritis may be useful in the chronic synovitis of psoriatic arthritis, although a convincing role for these agents has not yet been established. There is some evidence that gold can favourably affect the course of the arthritis and, in our experience, hydroxychloroquine has a similar effect. Sulphasalazine has recently been shown to be of benefit. D-penicillamine is not helpful.

        b. T—These drugs must be used with caution.

        c. F—Although it is true that the more severe cases of psoriasis are more likely to have an associated arthritis.

        d. T

        e. F—The same indications for intra-articular steroids apply as for rheumatoid arthritis. However, injecting into joints directly through psoriatic plaques is not advised since these plaques often harbour organisms such as *Staphylococcus aureus*. The use of systemic steroids in psoriatic arthritis is also inadvisable because of possible deterioration of the skin disease on stopping these drugs.

A.5.12 a. T

        b. T—The syndesmophytes of psoriatic spondylitis tend to be more patchy than in classical ankylosing spondylitis and have a somewhat "beaky" appearance and in this respect they are similar to those found in Reiter's syndrome.

        c. T

        d. T—This may be responsible for the well-known "pencil-in-cup" appearance of joints affected by psoriatic arthritis.

        e. F—Although spondylitis may affect the cervical spine, this usually leads to calcification of interspinous ligaments and apophyseal joints.

Q.5.13   Behçet's disease

    a. may cause blindness
    b. in males is associated with impotence
    c. is associated with a sterile pustular reaction to skin puncture
    d. is common in Japan
    e. may cause encephalitis
    f. all of the above
    g. none of the above

Q.5.14   Patients with Reiter's disease

    a. often have painful heels
    b. frequently have involvement of the small joints of the hand
    c. may suffer with recurrent iritis
    d. may have aortic incompetence
    e. commonly have a positive sheep cell agglutination test

Q.5.15   A male aged 20 years presents with an acutely painful swollen ankle. The following features may help in establishing a diagnosis:

    a. A positive family history of inflammatory bowel disease
    b. A history of recent travel abroad
    c. Therapy with erythromycin for acne vulgaris
    d. A pustular hyperkeratotic rash over the affected ankle
    e. A rash on the glans penis associated with a cheesy white exudate
    f. Employment in the leather industry

For answers see over

Answers

A.5.13 a. T—Due to anterior ocular inflammation (iritis) but more particularly posterior choroidoretinitis.

b. F—Although Behcet's disease may be associated with an epididymitis and scrotal ulcers.

c. T—This is otherwise known as skin hyper-reactivity or pathergy.

d. F—Behçet's disease is most frequently seen in Japan and the Mediterranean littoral but the maximum prevalence is still only 54 cases per 100 000 of the population.

e. T—And also a meningoencephalomyelitis.

f. F

g. F

A.5.14 a. T—Due to plantar fasciitis or an enthesitis where the Achilles tendon inserts into the calcaneum.

b. F—Usually large joints such as knee, wrist, ankle.

c. T

d. T

e. F

A.5.15 a. T—A positive family history of any of the seronegative arthritides may point to a diagnosis within this group of conditions.

b. T—A recent episode of dysentery may have precipitated post-dysenteric Reiter's syndrome.

c. F

d. T—This rash may be keratoderma blenorrhagica.

e. F—The rash described is suggestive of thrush due to *Candida albicans* and not circinate balanitis which would suggest Reiter's syndrome.

f. F

Q.5.16 The following gastro-intestinal diseases have been associated with a peripheral arthritis:

a. Coeliac disease
b. Regional ileitis (Crohn's disease)
c. Jejeuno-colostomy for morbid obesity
d. Diverticulosis coli
e. Multiple familial polyposis of the colon

Q.5.17 The following organisms have been implicated in the development of post-dysenteric reactive arthritis (Reiter's syndrome):

a. *Shigella flexneri*
b. *Salmonella typhi*
c. *Salmonella typhimurium*
d. *Campylobacter jejuni*
e. *Yersinia enterocolitica*
f. *All of the above*

Q.5.18 Sexually acquired reactive arthritis (Reiter's syndrome)

a. has a male preponderance
b. may follow infection with *Neisseria gonorrhoea*
c. has a good prognosis
d. responds to treatment with tetracycline
e. occurs more often in patients who are B27-positive

For answers see over

Answers

A.5.16 a. T—A seronegative symmetrical inflammatory polyarthritis has been reported in cases of coeliac disease. The arthritis is non-erosive and usually non-destructive.

b. T—A general asymmetrical large joint polyarthritis together with sacroiliitis and ankylosing spondylitis.

c. T—An asymmetrical polyarthritis which resolves on correction of the anatomical abnormality. It has been suggested that the arthritis results from immune complex deposition, the immune complexes arising from bacterial overgrowth in blind loops.

d. F

e. F

A.5.17 a. T

b. F

c. T

d. T

e. T

f. F

A.5.18 a. T—It may be that female Reiter's syndrome is not recognised because a female with a painful ankle is unlikely to have a vaginal examination for cervicitis.

b. T—In Reiter's syndrome *N. gonorrhoea* may be isolated from the genital tract but this may only be a co-infection with non-specific urethritis (in which other organisms, such as *Chlamydia trachomatis*, are implicated). In *N. gonorrhoea* septicaemia, generalised arthralgia may occur but, more usually, a true septic arthritis of one or more joints.

c. F—This became apparent on recent surveys where 83% of cases may still be suffering with polyarthritis over 5 years after the initial attack. Possibly this is due to reinfection.

d. F—If the original attack of Reiter's syndrome was precipitated by non-specific urethritis (probably due to chlamydia) then it is worth trying to eradicate this organism with a drug such as tetracycline. There is no evidence that this drug given at a later stage has a favourable outcome on the disease.

e. T—3% of those at risk, i.e., with non-specific urethritis, develop Reiter's syndrome; but 20% of those who are B27-positive develop the disease.

Q.5.19 In ankylosing spondylitis

   a. the disease is seen more frequently in males than females
   b. regular exercise prevents the progression of the disease
   c. problems may be encountered when driving
   d. sexual difficulties are uncommon
   e. there is an increased mortality due to pulmonary, renal and cardiac disease

Q.5.20 In the case of low back pain the following features suggest ankylosing spondylitis:

   a. Chronic low back pain, insidious in onset
   b. A male, aged less than 40 years
   c. Marked early morning stiffness
   d. Improvement of symptoms with exercise
   e. Sciatica

For answers see over

Answers

A.5.19 a. T—Although a survey of B27-positive blood donors in America found the ratio of male to female in this disease closer to unity. Possibly ankylosing spondylitis is less likely to be diagnosed in women because their symptoms are liable to be ignored or ascribed to pelvic problems.

b. T—Although this has never been shown in clinical trials. There is ample anecdotal evidence to show that if patients with ankylosing spondylitis are immobilised their spines rapidly fuse.

c. T—Because of cervical spine involvement so that special mirrors are needed for rear and side vision. Seat adaptations may also be necessary because of lumbar and thoracic spinal deformities.

d. F—In a recent survey, 50% of females and 20% of males reported sexual difficulties. The difference is probably explained by the males' reluctance to admit to sexual difficulties.

e. T—And this is independent of the treatment given. In cases that were treated by radiotherapy there is an increased incidence of neoplasia some 10–20 years later. In control cohorts not treated by radiation there is also an increased incidence of death due to gastrointestinal haemorrhage, presumably associated with anti-inflammatory drug treatment.

A.5.20 a. T
b. T
c. T
d. T
e. F

The group of symptoms listed in a-d has been shown to have an 85% sensitivity for diagnosing ankylosing spondylitis. Classical sciatica sometimes occurs in early ankylosing spondylitis. Some cases of ankylosing spondylitis are subjected to back surgery before the diagnosis is apparent.

Q.5.21 **The following are rarely found in psoriatic arthritis:**

   a. Involvement of the temporomandibular joints
   b. Bilateral sacroiliitis
   c. Arthritis mutilans
   d. Subcutaneous nodules
   e. Distal interphalangeal joint involvement
   f. Nail involvement
   g. Erosive disease on radiographic examination

Q.5.22 **A 50-year-old male with a 12-month history of polyarthritis is seen in the clinic. While taking a history you discover he has had recurrent attacks of iritis in the past. You would be alerted to the following conditions:**

   a. Sarcoidosis
   b. Gout
   c. Reiter's syndrome
   d. Ochronosis
   e. Ankylosing spondylitis
   f. Behçet's disease

Q.5.23 **A patient presents with arthritis and urethritis. In the differential diagnosis between gonorrhea and Reiter's syndrome the former is suggested by**

   a. conjunctivitis
   b. scanty white urethral discharge
   c. keratoderma blenorrhagica
   d. pharyngitis
   e. necrotic pustules on the hand

For answers see over

Answers

A.5.21 a. T
          b. F
          c. F
          d. T—If present, indicates rheumatoid arthritis.
          e. F—A classical presentation, usually with nail involvement.
          f. F
          g. F

A.5.22 a. T
          b. F
          c. T—Iritis occurs within the group of seronegative spondarthritides which includes Reiter's syndrome, ankylosing spondylitis, psoriatic arthritis and arthritis of inflammatory bowel disease.
          d. F—This may cause premature generalised osteoarthritis due to abnormal composition of cartilage.
          e. T
          f. T—Behçet's disease may cause iritis but also, and more importantly, causes a posterior choroidoretinitis. Behcet's disease is a major cause of blindness in Japan.

A.5.23 a. F—Except in congenital ophthalmnia neonatorum due to the gonococcus.
          b. F—May occur in both.
          c. F—Usually occurs in Reiter's syndrome.
          d. T—Positive throat swabs for gonococcus may occur in absence of symptoms.
          e. T—Septicaemia due to *N. gonorrhoea* may produce a generalised, discrete, erythematous, papular rash. These lesions may become necrotic and pustular.

Q.5.24 **Bilateral sacroiliitis may occur in**

    a. Reiter's syndrome
    b. psoriasis
    c. paraplegia
    d. juvenile chronic arthritis
    e. brucellosis
    f. all of the above

Q.5.25 **Calcaneal spurs are a recognised finding in**

    a. tertiary syphilis
    b. Reiter's syndrome
    c. fractures of the calcaneum
    d. Paget's disease of bone
    e. ankylosing spondylitis
    f. 25% of the population over the age of 50 years.

Q.5.26 **Pustulotic arthro-osteitis is characterised by**

    a. pustules on the palms and soles
    b. coincidental development of a peripheral arthritis
    c. uveitis
    d. involvement of the manubrio-sternal and sternoclavicular joints in a majority of cases
    e. spondylitis
    f. a good response to steroids

For answers see over

Answers

A.5.24 a. T

b. T—30% of patients with psoriatic arthritis have bilateral sacroiliitis.

c. F—An initial report suggested that sacroiliitis was common in paraplegia and that the likely cause was recurrent urinary tract infection causing sacroiliitis via lymphatic drainage. Subsequent reports, however, were unable to confirm this association by using strict radiological criteria.

d. T—In the patients who have a seronegative oligoarthritis (representing juvenile ankylosing spondylitis). However, radiographs of the sacroiliac joints are notoriously difficult to interpret in children.

e. F

f. F

A.5.25 a. F

b. T

c. F

d. F

e. T

f. T

Reiter's syndrome and ankylosing spondylitis belong to the group of seronegative spondarthritides. Plantar fasciitis can occur in both and calcification at the ligamentous insertions to the os calcis may subsequently develop. Asymptomatic plantar spurs in people over 50 years of age are generally smaller and do not exhibit associated erosive changes of the adjacent calcaneum.

A.5.26 a. T

b. T

c. F

d. T

e. T

f. F—These may exacerbate the pustulotic condition as in pustular psoriasis.

This condition has recently been described from Japan though some people believe this is a variant of psoriatic arthritis with associated spondylitis.

Q.5.27 **Assertion/Reason (p. vi):**

Statement 1 Anti-chlamydia antibodies are frequently found in cases of Reiter's disease

Statement 2 Chlamydia organisms can be isolated in 40% of cases of non-specific urethritis

Answer key:

Answer	First Statement	Second Statement	
a.	T	T	Second statement correctly explains first
b.	T	T	Second statement does *not* explain first
c.	T	F	
d.	F	T	
e.	F	F	

For answers see over

Answers

A.5.27 a. Anti-chlamydia antibodies are found in up to 36% of cases of Reiter's disease and these are likely to result from infection with *Chlamydia trachomatis* causing non-specific urethritis. Possibly other organisms will be implicated in future (such as *Yersinia* sp. from the gut).

6. Connective Tissue Disorders

Q.6.1   Characteristic associations of polyarteritis nodosa include

a. renal involvement in 80% of cases
b. aneurysm formation affecting medium-sized arteries
c. eosinophilia
d. positive Hb_SAg
e. abnormal C_3 level

Q.6.2   The following statements are true of lupus nephritis:

a. Clinical evidence of renal disease is present in over 70% of patients with SLE
b. The commonest histological lesion is membranoproliferative glomerulonephritis
c. C3 level in the serum may be a useful guide to disease activity
d. Exposure to sunlight may aggravate the severity
e. A deterioration in renal function may be due to renal vein thrombosis

Q.6.3   Adult dermatomyositis

a. deteriorates in pregnancy
b. produces proximal muscle wasting
c. may cause dysphagia
d. usually causes a deterioration in renal function
e. may be associated with upper lobe pulmonary fibrosis

Q.6.4   In drug-induced SLE

a. the onset is usually within the first week of starting the drug
b. peripheral arthritis is common
c. central nervous system involvement is typical
d. double-stranded DNA antibodies are present
e. rash is unusual

For answers see over

Answers

A.6.1 a. T—The commonest cause of death.
b. T—In diagnosis these are sought in the renal and coeliac circulation on angiography.
c. T
d. T—Without necessarily overt hepatitis.
e. F—Renal biopsy shows fibrin deposition but rarely C_3.

A.6.2 a. F—If sought, evidence of renal disease is present in about 50% of cases.
b. F—The commonest histological lesion is focal proliferative glomerulonephritis.
c. T—C3 may also be a useful guide to disease activity in general.
d. T—Patients with SLE and photosensitivity need appropriate warnings and should use high-factor sun-screen creams.
e. T—If a sudden deterioration in renal function occurs then appropriate investigation of this possibility must be sought.

A.6.3 a. T
b. F—Usually muscle weakness is much more evident than wasting.
c. T—But this may be late in the course of the disease.
d. F
e. F

A.6.4 a. F—Onset is usually related to cumulative dose of drug as with hydrallazine.
b. T—In 80%–90% of cases.
c. F—Also renal involvement is unusual.
d. F—Usually antibodies are to single-stranded DNA or histones.
e. F—Rash is not unusual.

Q.6.5   Giant cell (cranial) arteritis

a. may affect the popliteal artery
b. may cause a dissecting aneurysm of the aorta
c. may cause blindness
d. frequently affects patients under the age of 40 years
e. is associated with an elevated ESR
f. all of the above

Q.6.6   Henoch–Schönlein purpura (allergic leucocytoclastic vasculitis)

a. may follow infection with β-haemolytic Streptococcus
b. may be caused by penicillin
c. is associated with urticaria
d. may cause haemarthrosis
e. may cause splenomegaly

Q.6.7   In adult dermatomyositis

a. contracture of muscles rarely occurs early in the course of the disease
b. a heliotrope rash, consisting of purple raised macules on the face, is typical
c. myositis ossificans rarely occurs
d. antinuclear antibodies are rarely found
e. all of the above are true

For answers see over

Answers

A.6.5   a. T—Any medium-sized artery but usually the temporal artery, opthalmic artery and maxillary artery.

      b. F—The aortic arch syndrome, where several of the vessels coming off the aortic arch are affected by stenosing lesions at their origin, is seen in giant cell arteritis associated with Takayasu's disease.

      c. T

      d. F—This is extremely rare.

      e. T—Usually markedly elevated. In patients with a headache, tenderness of the temporal arteries and elevated ESR, steroids should be started prior to temporal artery biopsy because of the risk of blindness.

      f. F

A.6.6   a. T—May occasionally follow sore throat and infection with this organism.

      b. T

      c. F—The purpura of this condition is usually non-pruritic haemor-rhagic papules.

      d. F—But a synovitis of large joints may occur.

      e. F

A.6.7   a. T

      b. F—Heliotrope refers to the colour, lilac in hue, around the upper eyelids typical of this disease. Raised purple macules are more typical of discoid lupus.

      c. T—True myositis ossificans is rare but calcinosis can occur early in childhood cases and usually is deposited in the subcutaneous connective tissue and fascial planes. It may be severe enough to ulcerate through the skin and be extruded.

      d. T—Antinuclear antibodies are far more common in children than adults.

      e. F

Q.6.8 A "typical" rash is one of the diagnostic criteria for SLE. The following skin abnormalities may be found in SLE:

a. Alopecia
b. Vitiligo
c. Lupus pernio
d. Lupus vulgaris
e. Discoid lupus
f. Blistering photosensitivity

Q.6.9 Keratoconjunctivitis sicca occurs in

a. juvenile rheumatoid arthritis
b. Sjögren's syndrome
c. vitamin A deficiency
d. Reiter's syndrome
e. all of the above

Q.6.10 The following are true of CNS lupus:

a. C4 is always decreased in the cerebral spinal fluid
b. The patient usually has normal cerebral spinal fluid
c. The only abnormality in cerebral spinal fluid is a mild pleocytosis
d. Cranial neuropathies may occur
e. Psychosis may occur

Q.6.11 The following are found in nephrotic syndrome due to systemic lupus erythematosus:

a. Marked hypercholesterolaemia
b. Decreased serum complement
c. Red cells, white cells and granular casts
d. Focal proliferative glomerulonephritis on renal biopsy
e. Decreased creatinine clearance

For answers see over

Answers

A.6.8 a. T—Totalis or patchy alopecia may be present.
b. T—More often seen in negroes.
c. F—Lupus pernio occurs in sarcoidosis.
d. F—The rash used to describe cutaneous tuberculosis (formerly known as scrofula).
e. T—Although only a small percentage go on to develop SLE.
f. T—Photosensitivity is acknowledged as a typical SLE rash.

A.6.9 a. F—Chronic insidious iridocyclitis is the usual ocular manifestation.
b. T
c. T
d. F—More usually uveitis or iritis is the ocular complication.
e. F

A.6.10 a. F
b. T
c. T
d. T
e. T

Although the CSF is usually normal in cases of CNS lupus, occasionally a mild leucocytosis is found but complement levels show little change. Psychosis is the most common psychiatric manifestation of CNS lupus. Generalised fits may also occur. Localised CNS lupus may cause peripheral neuropathy, transverse myelitis and chorea.

A.6.11 a. F—Marked hypercholesterolaemia is an uncommon manifestation of the nephrotic syndrome due to SLE.
b. T
c. T
d. T—However other histological findings may occur and these include membranous glomerulonephritis, membrano proliferative glomerulonephritis and diffuse proliferative glomerulonephritis. None of these appearances are characteristic.
e. T

Q.6.12   Assertion/Reason (see p. vi):

   Statement 1   In SLE antigen/antibody complexes of DNA/
   IgG are found on the glomerular basement
   membrane

   Statement 2   Disease activity in SLE is proportional to DNA
   binding (measured by the Farr assay)

   Answer key:

Answer	First statement	Second statement	
a.	T	T	Second statement correctly explains first
b.	T	T	Second statement does *not* explain first
c.	T	F	
d.	F	T	
e.	F	F	

Q.6.13   A 23-year-old female is admitted with a diffuse erythematous non-pruritic rash over her face and a temperature of 38.5°C. She has had episodes of leucopenia in the past and is now taking procainamide for a cardiac arrhythmia. DNA binding is 45% by the Farr technique; urinalysis reveals numerous red cell casts; there is 2.5 g protein in the urine in 24 h. The following are true:

   a. The patient has naturally occurring systemic lupus erythematosus
   b. Because of her anti-DNA antibodies, one cannot differentiate between naturally occurring and drug-induced SLE
   c. Serum complement would be of value
   d. The patient should be treated with immunosuppressives
   e. Procainamide should be stopped

For answers see over

Answers

A.6.12 c. Although a direct pathogenetic mechanism for anti-nuclear antibody in SLE has not yet been proven, circumstantial evidence (e.g., antigen/antibody complexes in the kidney) is suggestive. However, other evidence, notably that antinuclear factors may cross the placenta without causing damage to the foetus (the exception to this are Ro and La antibodies), would suggest otherwise. In addition lupus plasma has been transfused into non-lupus patients without harmful effect. The serum level of C3, not the % DNA binding, is a more useful guide to disease activity.

A.6.13 a. T—Drug-induced SLE is rarely complicated by renal disease and antibodies to native DNA are rarely found.
b. F—Procainamide-induced SLE is usually associated with anti-histone antibodies.
c. T—In naturally occurring SLE with renal disease the serum complement level is a useful guide to disease activity.
d. F—Steroids are usually the first-choice drug for renal complications of SLE.
e. F

Q.6.14 **The following statements about the cutaneous manifestations of SLE are true:**

    a. An abnormality of the skin, hair or mucous membranes is one of the commonest manifestations of SLE

    b. Alopecia may be localised or diffuse

    c. Photosensitivity may be exacerbated by treatment with chloroquine

    d. Patients with plaques characterised by hyperkeratosis, follicular plugging and subsequent scarring usually have antibodies to native DNA

    e. Osler's nodes may be found

Q.6.15 **The arthritis of SLE may**

    a. resemble that of rheumatoid arthritis with the presence of symmetrical soft tissue swelling of the proximal interphalangeal joints

    b. be associated with subcutaneous nodules over bony prominences

    c. rarely causes radiological erosive change in the joints

    d. be associated with correctable deformity of the joints (Jaccoud's arthritis)

    e. usually be helped by treatment with non-steroidal anti-inflammatory drugs

Q.6.16 **In SLE the heart may be affected in the following manner:**

    a. An asymptomatic pericardial effusion is present in the majority of cases

    b. Pericardial tamponade rarely occurs

    c. Verrucous-like endocardial vegetations may cause a cardiac murmur

    d. There is an increased incidence of sudden death due to myocardial infarction

    e. Where a cardiac murmur is present, appropriate precautions to prevent sub-acute bacterial endocarditis must be taken

For answers see over

Answers

A.6.14 a. T—90% have fever, 85% have skin changes.
       b. T
       c. T
       d. F—The description is of chronic discoid lupus erythematosus of which less than 10% progress to systemic lupus erythematosus. Antibodies to DNA are found in the minority.
       e. T—Due to small areas of vasculitis in the skin. Tender nodular lesions in the palm are called Janeway lesions.

A.6.15 a. T—Initial appearance may be identical. Beware the confusion of overlap syndromes where patients with rheumatoid arthritis are anti-nuclear antibody positive and have other features of SLE, such as Raynaud's phenomenon.
       b. F—Subcutaneous nodules over bony prominences associated with symmetrical arthritis are the hallmark of rheumatoid arthritis.
       c. T
       d. T—Originally used to describe the appearance of the joints following rheumatic fever; another cause of "Jaccoud's arthritis" is hypermobility.
       e. T

A.6.16 a. F—Echocardiographic studies have revealed asymptomatic pericardial effusion in 30% of cases of SLE.
       b. T—This occurs rarely, but patients are at definite risk from this complication due to the development of a large effusion.
       c. F—Verrucous-like endocardial vegetations are present pathologically in nearly all cases and do not correlate with murmurs. With scarring, overt aortic incompetence or mitral incompetence may occur.
       d. T—But this complication is usually seen in steroid-treated younger subjects possibly having coronary arteritis.
       e. T

Q.6.17 **Anticardiolipin antibodies**

a. are the cause of a false-positive test for syphilis
b. may be determined indirectly by an estimation of the pro-thrombin time
c. are associated with vascular thrombosis in SLE
d. may be associated with recurrent miscarriage
e. are responsible for cardiac conduction defects

Q.6.18 **The following statements are true:**

a. Antinuclear factor is present in 30% of cases of seropositive rheumatoid arthritis
b. Ro and La are components of the cell membrane
c. Antibodies to double stranded (native) DNA are detectable by employing the protozoon *Crithidia lucidae*
d. DNA binding is a measure of the affinity of autologous IgG for labelled DNA, and is expressed as a percentage of the maximum
e. In drug-induced SLE antibodies to histones are frequently found
f. None of the above

Q.6.19 **While on call one Friday night you receive a telephone call from an anxious psychiatric Registrar at a neighbouring hospital. One week ago they admitted a 20-year-old female with symptoms suggesting schizophrenia, but her conscious level has suddenly deteriorated. The only other significant features are a history of photosensitivity and what he describes as a right central retinal vein thrombosis on fundoscopy. You arrange transfer. CNS lupus is suspected. The following are correct:**

a. SLE may present as a psychiatric illness
b. Unilateral haemorrhages and exudates visible on fundoscopy are always due to central retinal vein thrombosis
c. Neuroradiology may help
d. Anticardiolipin antibodies are invariably present in CNS lupus
e. Treatment with high-dose steroids is urgently indicated if CNS lupus is suspected

For answers see over

Answers

A.6.17 a. T—Reagin, the antigen used, is an acid phospholipid similar to cardiolipin.

b. F—Usually the activated partial thromboplastin time (APTT) is used as an indirect measure of "lupus anticoagulant". Despite an increased tendency to vascular thrombosis there is a paradoxical prolongation of the APTT due to the anticardiolipin antibodies. This in vitro clotting abnormality is not correctable by the addition of serum from a healthy person.

c. T

d. T—Possibly due to placental infarction. There may be no relation to SLE in these subjects.

e. F—Antibodies to nuclear antigen Ro(SSA) have been implicated in congenital heart block.

A.6.18 a. F—Antinuclear factor is present in 10%–15% of cases of rheumatoid arthritis, probably less in males.

b. F—Ro and La are extractable nuclear antigens.

c. T

d. T

e. T—Anti-DNA antibodies are usually negative.

f. F

A.6.19 a. T

b. F—Retinal vasculitis may present a similar picture.

c. T—Cerebral infarction may be apparent on enhanced CT scans. Magnetic resonance imaging may show a diffuse abnormality in CNS lupus. CT scanning may also help to exclude other causes of cerebral obtundation such as tumour.

d. F—Cerebral vasculitis is not associated with anticardiolipin antibodies although cerebral thrombosis is linked.

e. T—Anticoagulants may also be necessary if thrombotic events are suspected.

Q.6.20   Antinuclear antibody negative SLE

    a. may occur if HEp 2 cells are used instead of mouse liver slices for detection of antinuclear factor

    b. may occur if antinuclear antibody is present in very high titre

    c. may occur where heavy proteinuria is present

    d. where genuinely negative is associated with a better prognosis

    e. may be associated with anti-Ro antibodies

Q.6.21   Dermatomyositis

    a. is always associated with underlying malignancy

    b. causes bulbar weakness in the early stages

    c. typically presents with a rash on the extensor aspects of the joints

    d. frequently leads to muscle contractures

    e. causes subcutaneous calcinosis

    f. may cause cardiac conduction abnormalities

Q.6.22   Match the following:

    a. CREST syndrome

    b. Eosinophilic fasciitis

    c. Morphoea

    d. Progressive systemic sclerosis

    e. Dermatomyositis

    A. May be precipitated by a period of unaccustomed exertion

    B. Circumscribed areas of fibrosis involving the skin and sub-cutaneous tissue

    C. May be associated with underlying malignancy

    D. May cause dysphagia

    E. Anticentromere antibodies frequently present

For answers see over

Answers

A.6.20 a. F—HEp 2 cells are a more sensitive indicator of antinuclear antibody.
      b. T
      c. T—Because the antibody may leak out into the urine.
      d. T—Usually there is a high incidence of photosensitivity but a low incidence of renal and neuropsychiatric complications.
      e. T—These may not be apparent on immunofluorescence.

A.6.21 a. F—If the patient is over 40 years of age then over half the casts are associated with an underlying malignancy, usually stomach or breast.
      b. F—But this may be a late feature.
      c. T—These are called Goddron's patches and consist of scaly erythematous plaques. In addition, a typical heliotrope (lilac hue) rash occurs on the eyelids and periorbital area.
      d. T—And these need to be prevented by appropriate physiotherapy.
      e. T—Especially in children.
      f. T—Congestive cardiac failure may also occur.

A.6.22 a. E
      b. A
      c. B
      d. D
      e. C

Q.6.23 Systemic sclerosis is a difficult disease to treat. The following assertions are true:

    a. D-penicillamine is used because of its in vitro ability to prevent abnormal cross-linkage formation in collagen

    b. Beta-blockers are useful in the treatment.of hypertension due to renal disease

    c. Colchicine has been shown to prevent collagen formation in vitro

    d. Potassium aminobenzoic acid (POTABA) is a useful treatment because it increases tissue oxygen

    e. The only effective treatment for pulmonary fibrosis is systemic steroids

Q.6.24 The following can occur as neuro-psychiatric features of systemic lupus erythematosus and may respond to treatment of the SLE:

    a. Schizophrenia
    b. Depression
    c. Grand mal fits
    d. Devic's syndrome
    e. Peripheral neuropathy
    f. Myasthenia gravis
    g. All of these
    h. None of these

For answers see over

Answers

A.6.23 a. F—Although clinical trials have been disappointing with this
drug, possibly because collagen changes in skin and other
organs are already advanced at the time of diagnosis.

b. F—Beta-blockers are best avoided because they may exacerbate Raynaud's phenomenon which is a feature of the
disease.

c. T—But the same considerations apply as with D-penicillamine.

d. F—POTABA has been used in the treatment of scleroderma
following in vitro evidence that it caused an increase in tissue
oxygen concentration and, since many of the changes in
scleroderma were thought to be ischaemic in origin. Controlled
trials of POTABA in scleroderma have not been performed.

e. F—There is no effective treatment for the pulmonary fibrosis
due to systemic sclerosis.

A.6.24 a. T

b. T

c. T

d. T

e. T

f. T

g. T

h. F

Q.6.25 A 30-year-old female with a history of a photosensitive rash, leucopenia and strongly positive antinuclear factor (homogeneous pattern) presents with heavy proteinuria. The figure represents the appearances of a glomerulus as seen by light microscopy on renal biopsy specimens. The following statements are true:

a. Clinical evidence of renal involvement occurs in all subjects with SLE at some time
b. The appearances indicate a good prognosis
c. Immunofluorescent microscopy will add little additional information
d. The patient should be given high dose oral steroids
e. The patient should be advised to avoid sun-bathing

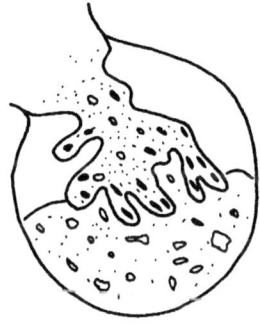

For answers see over

Answers

A.6.25   a. F—Pathological evidence of renal involvement on renal biopsy is present in the majority of cases.

b. F—The appearances indicate diffuse proliferative glomerular nephritis with crescent formation. Whereas the proliferative pattern occurs in the majority of cases of SLE, membranous and mesangial proliferation may also occur. When appearances are diffuse the prognosis is poor.

c. T—Although IgG and complement may be demonstrated lining the basement membrane.

d. T—Some centres would give high dose intravenous steroids with additional pulses of cyclophosphamide. Plasmapheresis is of unproven value.

e. T—The renal disease may be exacerbated by development of a photosensitive rash. If light exposure is necessary then a high factor sun screen should be used.

7. Soft Tissue Rheumatism and Regional Pain Syndromes

Q.7.1   Capsulitis of the shoulder ("frozen shoulder")

a. occurs more frequently in diabetics
b. usually resolves spontaneously in 6–9 months
c. may be precipitated by trauma
d. causes a painful arc on active shoulder abduction
e. frequently causes sleep disturbance
f. rarely occurs bilaterally

Q.7.2   This statement is true of polymyalgia rheumatica:

a. Most patients are over the age of 50 years
b. About 25% of patients develop unilateral or bilateral blindness
c. The response to steroids is often so dramatic that patients are markedly improved after one or two tablets
d. CPK is often elevated
e. All of the above

Q.7.3   In spinal claudication

a. symptoms are typically worse when the patient walks downhill
b. examination may be entirely normal
c. a plain X-ray film of the lumbo-sacral spine may be normal
d. signs may develop after exercise on a bicycle ergometer
e. the condition frequently co-exists with other evidence of arterial disease

For answers see over

Answers

A.7.1 a. T—May also occur on the hemiplegic side following stroke, and after coronary thrombosis.

        b. F—The pain rarely subsides in less than a year and may be persistent for up to two years. Following resolution of the pain, shoulder movements are still restricted.

        c. T

        d. F—A painful arc on shoulder abduction is characteristic of a rotator cuff lesion. Typically, in capsulitis patients cannot abduct their shoulder above 90° and all shoulder movements both active and passive are painful.

        e. T—This may cause amplification of the pain in the shoulder. For this reason it is important to treat this symptom seriously.

        f. T—It is unusual for capsulitis to occur bilaterally at the same time.

A.7.2 a. T

        b. F—Blindness is a complication of temporal arteritis which occurs in association with polymyalgia. Any patient with symptoms of polymyalgia and headaches should be suspected of having temporal arteritis and, because of the risk of blindness, steroids should be started immediately. Steroid treatment will not affect biopsy evidence of temporal arteritis providing this is performed within a short period of starting these drugs.

        c. T—Often the patient wakes up the next morning almost cured of symptoms.

        d. F—Muscle enzymes, EMG and muscle biopsy are usually normal.

        e. F

A.7.3 a. T—Walking downhill involves extension of the lumbar spine, which reduces the diameter of the spinal canal. Conversely, flexion of the lumbar spine increases the spinal canal diameter and patients with spinal claudication comment that bending forward relieves their pain.

        b. T—Although signs may be precipitated by exercise.

        c. T—Often CT or ultrasound scan are necessary to diagnose this condition.

        d. F

        e. F—It is the spinal canal diameter and not the state of the arterial tree which is critical.

Q.7.4 A useful treatment in capsulitis of the shoulder is

a. high-dose oral steroids
b. non-steroidal anti-inflammatory drugs
c. physiotherapy
d. manipulation under anaesthetic
e. intra-articular steroids
f. all of the above

Q.7.5 Assertion/Reason (see p. vi):

Statement 1 Low back pain is a common symptom in middle age
Statement 2 The prevalence of degenerative lumbar spondylosis increases with age

Answer key:

Answer	First statement	Second statement	
a.	T	T	Second statement correctly explains first
b.	T	T	Second statement does *not* explain first
c.	T	F	
d.	F	T	
e.	F	F	

For answers see over

Answers

A.7.4   a. T
        b. T
        c. T
        d. T
        e. T
        f. T

Although all of the above treatments have been claimed to be of use, in fact the condition is often refractory to any form of treatment. Eventual spontaneous resolution usually occurs. In the acutely painful stage adequate analgesia is required, if necessary using non-steroidae anti-inflammatory drugs. When the pain diminishes, physiotherapy is recommended to restore the range of movement. Some European physicians use high-dose oral steroids initially. It is possible that if capsulitis is seen and treated in its early stages by intra-articular steroids then this treatment may be effective in shortening the natural history, but this suggestion awaits confirmation.

A.7.5   b. It is difficult to make a direct link between low back pain and degenerative lumbar spondylosis since degenerative spondylosis is seen equally in people presenting with other conditions unrelated to the back. The diagnostic yield of plain lumbar radiography in cases of clinical mechanical low back pain is virtually nil for this reason and unless there are good clinical reasons (for example, persistent pain including nocturnal pain, fever, weight loss and other constitutional symptoms, or a specific history of carcinoma or infection elsewhere) plain radiography is usually unhelpful.

Q.7.6 **Match the following:**

 a. Golfer's elbow
 b. Tennis elbow
 c. Miner's elbow
 d. Baker's cyst
 e. Housemaid's knee
 f. Clergyman's knee

 A. Enlarged semi-membranosus bursa
 B. Infra-patellar bursitis
 C. Olecranon bursitis
 D. Lateral epicondylitis
 E. Pre-patellar bursitis
 F. Medial epicondylitis

Q.7.7 **Patients with repetitive strain injury**

 a. are eligible to receive Industrial Injuries Disablement Benefit
 b. may be eligible for a pension as a result of contracting an occupational disease
 c. may not continue their employment if in receipt of Industrial Injuries Disablement Benefit or a pension
 d. are the leading cause of compensatable injury in the UK
 e. may be dismissed by their employer despite acquiring the disability in that employment

Q.7.8 **Repetitive strain injury**

 a. may be associated with definite adverse histological changes in the affected muscles
 b. is a notifiable disease
 c. may result in Sudek's atrophy
 d. may cause osteoarthritis
 e. requires objective clinical signs for diagnosis

For answers see over

Answers

A.7.6 a. F
        b. D
        c. C
        d. A
        e. E
        f. B

A Baker's cyst may be due to an enlarged semi-membranosus or gastrocnemius bursa, either of which may communicate with the knee joint.

A.7.7 a. T—Although this only occurs rarely as this benefit is paid only if injury can be shown to be due to an accident while employed.
        b. T—Although the level of disability at which this pension may be paid has been arbitrarily fixed at 14%.
        c. F
        d. F—Repetitive strain injury is the second cause, the most common cause being pneumoconiosis.
        e. T

A.7.8 a. T—Lancet (1988) 1:905.
        b. F
        c. T
        d. F
        e. F—Symptoms are sufficient.

Repetitive strain injury is a relatively new and fashionable diagnosis which has recently reached epidemic proportions in Australia. The spectrum of this disorder covers anything from repetitive damage to the joint causing osteoarthritis through tenosynovitis to myalgia following extended working periods.

Q.7.9   The tarsal tunnel syndrome

a. may occur in hypothyroidism
b. causes pain and paraesthesiae on the medial aspect of the dorsum of the foot
c. is due to entrapment of the common peroneal nerve
d. may be treated by an injection of steroid into the tarsal tunnel just lateral to the tendon of extensor hallucis longus at the ankle
e. does not exist!

Q.7.10   In primary fibromyalgia (generalised non-articular rheumatism)

a. sleep disturbance may be severe
b. muscle enzymes are occasionally elevated
c. patients are often intolerant of non-steroidal anti-inflammatory drugs
d. the condition may be precipitated by an injury
e. there is an association with spastic colon (irritable bowel syndrome)

Q.7.11   The following abnormalities are typical of polymyalgia rheumatica:

a. Wasted shoulder and hip girdle muscles
b. Positive sheep cell agglutination test
c. Abnormal electromyography
d. CPK elevation
e. Positive family history

Q.7.12   The following are signs of supraspinatus tendinitis:

a. A painful arc on active abduction of the shoulder
b. Painful resisted internal rotation of the shoulder
c. Full passive range of shoulder movement
d. Tenderness antero-lateral to the acromion
e. Limited passive gleno-humoral abduction

For answers see over

Answers

A.7.9 a. F
  b. F
  c. F
  d. F
  e. F—This condition is rarely diagnosed by some rheumatologists but is often seen by others. The symptoms are pain and para-esthesae on the medial aspect of the sole of the foot due to entrapment of the posterior tibial nerve underneath the fibrous band connecting the medial malleolus with the medial aspect of the calcaneum. It may be relieved by an injection of steroid into the tarsal tunnel just inferior to the medial malleolus.

A.7.10 a. T—This is thought to contribute to the syndrome.
  b. F
  c. T—Patients often consider themselves allergic to foodstuffs and other drugs as well.
  d. T—The condition may be considered an inappropriate neuro-physiological response to this injury.
  e. T

A.7.11 a. F
  b. F
  c. F
  d. F
  e. F
  None of these are found in classical polymyalgia rheumatica. Usually there are no objective signs of muscle wasting or EMG abnormalities and CPK is normal. There is no evidence of familial association. The presence of positive serology is controversial since often rheumatoid arthritis may start with a polymyalgic-like syndrome and recently cases of polymyalgia have been reported to occur in patients with rheumatoid arthritis.

A.7.12 a. T
  b. F—This is more typical of subscapularis tendinitis.
  c. T
  d. T—At the insertion of the tendon.
  e. F—All passive movements of the shoulder should be normal, although on occasion pain is elicited in the shoulder at the limit of gleno-humeral abduction as the tendon is trapped under the acromion.

Q.7.13 **Anterior knee joint pain is a common complaint in adolescents referred to hospital. Chondomalacia patella is a frequent diagnostic label. The following statements are true:**

    a. Untreated, the prognosis is good
    b. The clinical picture is characteristic
    c. Arthroscopy may be necessary for diagnosis
    d. The characteristic findings on arthroscopy are fibrillation and erosion of articular cartilage of the medial facet of the patella
    e. Chondromalacia patella is a normal finding
    f. All of the above

Q.7.14 **The following are recognised examples of referred pain:**

    a. Pain in the shoulder originating from the cervical spine
    b. Pain in the elbow arising from the shoulder
    c. Pain in the posterior thigh arising from the hip
    d. Pain in the knee arising from the hip
    e. Pain in the central abdomen arising from the lumbar spine

Q.7.15 **Subjective swelling and stiffness of the joints are frequent complaints in musculoskeletal disorders. The following statements are true:**

    a. Enlargement of the joint may be due to bone or synovial hypertrophy
    b. Carpal tunnel syndrome frequently causes subjective swelling of the hand
    c. Prolonged early morning stiffness is a feature of osteoarthritis
    d. In rheumatoid arthritis, joint stiffness is related to the extent of joint destruction by the disease
    e. Transient swelling of a joint is a feature of gout

For answers see over

Answers

A.7.13   a. T
b. T—Anterior knee pain in an adolescent with retropatellar crepitus and pain elicited when the patella is compressed against the femur.
c. T
d. T
e. T
f. T

Although chondromalacia patella is frequently diagnosed clinically there is some uncertainty as to the relevance of the macroscopic retropatellar abnormalities. These abnormalities have been seen in asymptomatic knees and are only present in 50% of knees with the clinical syndrome.

A.7.14   a. T
b. T
c. F—Usually anterior thigh.
d. T
e. F—Central abdominal pain may be due to referred pain from the lower thoracic spine.

A.7.15   a. T—This is a basic distinction to be made when examining joints in order to assess the presence of an inflammatory arthropathy.
b. T
c. F—Early morning stiffness may occur in osteoarthritis but is usually of short duration.
d. F—joint stiffness in rheumatoid arthritis is most pronounced in the early stages and may be minimal when subluxation of the joint has occurred. Objective measures of stiffness do not confirm the patients' impression and possibly patients mistake pain for stiffness in inflammatory arthritis.
e. T

Q.7.16 In cervical spondylosis

a. passive movements of the neck often exceed active movements

b. there may be no symptoms

c. torticollis frequently occurs

d. chronic nerve root pain is uncommon

e. compression of the C5 nerve root leads to a reduced supinator jerk

Q.7.17 In the management of acute lumbago

a. radiology of the lumbo-sacral spine is unhelpful

b. manipulation produces long-term results consistently better than any other treatment

c. bed-rest is not of proven benefit

d. 90% of cases recover by one month

e. muscle relaxants are an essential part of the treatment

Q.7.18 A 70-year-old patient with persistently active rheumatoid arthritis has been started on prednisolone and azathioprine. Four months later her disease is less active but she presents in the casualty department with severe pain in the distribution marked in the figure. X-ray examination shows a discitis at L4/L5. Possible management strategies include

a. bed-rest and traction

b. needle aspiration biopsy of the L4/5 disc

c. treatment with oral acyclovir

d. X-ray examination of cervical spine in flexion and extension

e. reduction in dose of prednisolone and azathioprine

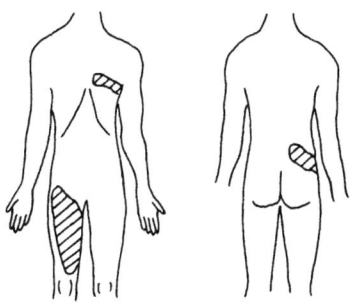

For answers see over

Answers

A.7.16
a. F
b. T—The majority of cervical spines in people over the age of 50 years show some degenerative change.
c. F
d. T
e. F—Compression of C5 root causes reduction in biceps jerk.

A.7.17
a. T
b. F—Manipulation has been shown to give early relief of pain but the long-term results are similar to other methods of treatment.
c. F—Bed-rest for 2–5 days is more effective at relieving pain than ambulatory treatment.
d. T
e. F—Nor has objective evidence for muscle spasm been obtained.

A.7.18
a. F—Although the distribution of the pain in the back and leg is compatible with L2 nerve root irritation, this root is rarely involved by a prolapsed intravertebral disc.
b. F—Discitis can occur as a complication of rheumatoid arthritis. In the absence of systemic symptoms or radiological evidence of progression and associated bone destruction, infection is unlikely.
c. T—The distribution of pain in the L2 and T4 nerve roots is highly suggestive of a sensory radiculopathy due to *Herpes zoster* virus.
d. F
e. T—Since these drugs, by virtue of their immunosuppressive properties, probably precipitated the *H. zoster* infection.

Q.7.19 **A 75-year-old female complains of severe neck and shoulder pain. The following findings would help confirm a diagnosis of polymyalgia rheumatica:**

a. Marked shoulder girdle muscle tenderness
b. Loss of weight and fever
c. Proteinuria
d. Positive muscle biopsy
e. Dramatic and early response to oral steroid therapy

For answers see over

Answers

A.7.19   a. T—The pelvic girdle may also be involved.

            b. T—Systemic symptoms are occasionally prominent and, as well as loss of weight and fever, include depression.

            c. F

            d. F

            e. T—Treatment is usually continued for at least 12 months and is often necessary for up to two years. The minimum dose of steroid necessary to control symptoms should be used.

8. Crystal Disease and Osteoarthritis

Q.8.1 **Recognised features of generalised osteoarthritis include**

a. Clutton's joints
b. Schmorl's nodes
c. Heberden's nodes
d. Bouchard's nodes
e. Romanus lesions

Q.8.2 **The following metabolic conditions may predispose to osteoarthritis:**

a. Simple morbid obesity
b. Hyperthyroidism
c. Diabetes mellitus
d. Type 1 glycogen storage disease
e. Acromegaly
f. Haemochromatosis

Q.8.3 **The following statements are true about changes seen radiographically in osteoarthritis:**

a. Calcium pyrophosphate deposition is common
b. Marginal erosions are common
c. Joint space narrowing reflects cartilage loss
d. Clinical symptoms do not correlate with radiological progress
e. Improvement in radiological appearance may occur.

For answers see over

Answers

A.8.1   a.   F—Clutton's joints result from congenital syphilis and present in childhood, occasionally mimicking juvenile chronic arthritis of the knees. Treatment is entirely symptomatic and diagnosis depends on identifying other features of congenital syphilis.

          b.   F—These are herniation of disc material into the end plate of adjacent vertebrae.

          c.   T—Heberden's nodes are essentially osteophytes on the joint margin of the distal interphalangeal joints.

          d.   T—Marginal osteophytes on the proximal interphalangeal joints of the fingers.

          e.   F—Romanus lesions are erosions on the anterior/superior border of the upper lumbar and lower thoracic vertebrae seen in early ankylosing spondylitis.

A.8.2   a.   T—Epidemiologically, there is an association between "severe" morbid obesity and osteoarthritis and this pertains not only to weight-bearing joints but to joints such as the distal interphalangeal joints. Possibly there is an associated metabolic defect that predisposes to obesity and premature cartilage degeneration.

          b.   F—Although hypothyroidism does.

          c.   F—Associated conditions are Charcot's joints, DISH, capsulitis of shoulder and cheiroarthropathy.

          d.   F

          e.   T—There is overgrowth of abnormal cartilage and premature degeneration of the joint.

          f.   T—Calcium pyrophosphate deposition may be associated with consequent degenerative change.

A.8.3   a.   T—Increasing with age and not necessarily causing acute pseudo-gout.

          b.   F—More likely in inflammatory arthritis such as rheumatoid.

          c.   T

          d.   T

          e.   T—Some people suggest that healing may occur with regeneration of cartilage in occasional cases.

Q.8.4 **The following remarks are true of osteoarthritis:**

a. Thin people do not suffer from it
b. The ankle joint is not usually affected
c. The degree of pain is a good indication of the amount of damage to the joint
d. Pain is typically worse after the joint has been in use
e. There is now good evidence that non-steroidal anti-inflammatory drugs help joint healing in addition to relieving pain.

Q.8.5 **Osteoarthritis**

a. characteristically begins at about the age of 50 years
b. is three times more common in men
c. is commonest in the hip
d. is not predominantly an inflammatory condition
e. gives pain that is worse in the evening
f. does not cause morning stiffness

Q.8.6 **A male aged 40 years presents with unilateral hip pain. X-ray examination reveals extensive osteoarthritis of the hip. Other joints are normal and he is otherwise well. The following conditions could have caused this history:**

a. Sickle-cell disease
b. Slipped upper femoral epiphysis
c. Congenital dislocation of the hip
d. Gout
e. Perthes' disease

For answers see over

Answers

A.8.4 a. F—However, obesity may aggravate the symptoms in weight-bearing joints. Obesity is linked in animals and, in some studies, humans to osteoarthritis and may reflect a metabolic defect common to both.

b. T

c. F—Radiological damage does not correlate with clinical symptoms. Symptoms may be severe with little change and vice versa.

d. T

e. F—There is a claim that some non-steroidal anti-inflammatory drugs are now chondroprotective, that is, they do not have any adverse effects on chondrocyte function in vitro. However, there is no evidence that this is relevant clinically. It is, in fact, possible that non-steroidal anti-inflammatory drugs may permit increased joint damage to occur because of their analgesic effects. Some reports have suggested non-steroidal anti-inflammatory drugs may cause avascular necrosis of the hip, presumably by compromising the blood supply to this area, although no controlled studies have confirmed this.

A.8.5 a. T—It is very unusual in younger age groups unless there is a predisposing cause such as an inflammatory arthritis, a congenital or acquired deformity, or a metabolic abnormality of cartilage.

b. F—It is three times more common in women.

c. F—The knees and hands are the commonest sites.

d. T—Unlike, for example, rheumatoid arthritis. However, synovial biopsies have revealed a low grade inflammatory exudate in these osteoarthritic joints but the clinical significance of this is doubtful.

e. T—Especially after using the joint heavily during the day.

f. T—This may occur, but usually it is only of short duration (less than 30 minutes). Typically patients also experience articular gelling (brief inactivity stiffness).

A.8.6 a. T—Due to avascular necrosis of the femoral head.

b. T

c. T

d. F

e. T

Q.8.7 In the elderly, osteoarthritis is commonly seen in the following joints:

a. Knee
b. Ankle (tibio-talar)
c. Trapezio-metacarpal
d. Elbow
e. Apophyseal

Q.8.8 Assertion/Reason (see p. vi):

Statement 1   Non-steroidal anti-inflammatory drugs are effective in relieving symptoms in osteoarthritis

Statement 2   The histology of the synovial tissue in osteoarthritis frequently shows inflammatory cells

Answer key:

Answer	First statement	Second statement	
a.	T	T	Second statement correctly explains first
b.	T	T	Second statement does *not* explain first
c.	T	F	
d.	F	T	
e.	F	F	

For answers see over

Answers

A.8.7   a. T
          b. F
          c. T
          d. F
          e. T

Epidemiological studies have shown an exponential rise in radiological osteoarthritis with age. The commonly affected joints are the knee, hip, distal interphalangeal of the fingers, the trapeziometacarpal joints, the apophyseal and the intervertebral joints. Note that not only weight-bearing joints are affected and note also that only a few percent of cases surveyed radiologically in the community are symptomatic.

A.8.8   b. The degree of inflammation seen in osteoarthritic synovium is much less than that seen in inflammatory arthritides such as rheumatoid arthritis. Simple analgesics are often as effective as anti-inflammatory drugs in this condition and it is likely that in the majority of cases, anti-inflammatory drugs are acting as pure analgesics in relieving pain. Occasionally, where acute crystal synovitis supervenes or where there is evidence of more significant inflammation clinically, the specific anti-inflammatory effect of non-steroidal anti-inflammatory drugs may be needed.

Q.8.9   Assertion/Reason (see p. vi):

Statement 1   Hypermobility is much more prevalent in females than males

Statement 2   Osteoarthritis is predominantly a disease of postmenopausal females

Answer key:

Answer	First statement	Second statement	
a.	T	T	Second statement correctly explains first
b.	T	T	Second statement does *not* explain first
c.	T	F	
d.	F	T	
e.	F	F	

Q.8.10   In osteoarthritis

a. hydrarthrosis of more than one joint at a time is uncommon
b. osteoporosis and soft tissue atrophy are typical
c. subluxation of the joint does not occur
d. narrowing of the cartilage space is typically non-uniform
e. co-existing crystal arthropathy is not unusual

Q.8.11   Allopurinol

a. may potentiate the hypoglycaemic action of chlorpropamide
b. may precipitate gout
c. may be given intermittently
d. may cause thrombocytopenic purpura
e. may usefully be combined with probenecid

For answers see over

Answers

A.8.9 b. As yet, it has not been shown that there is a causal association between generalised hypermobility and generalised osteoarthritis although isolated hypermobility has been linked to subsequent osteoarthritis in that joint. Possibly there is a shared metabolic defect causing the two conditions but this has not yet been shown.

A.8.10 a. T

       b. F—It has been suggested that osteoporosis and osteoarthrosis rarely co-exist. Conversely, patients with Paget's disease encroaching upon the joint surface often have accelerated osteoarthritic changes.

       c. T—This is more typical of an inflammatory arthritis where the collateral ligaments are weakened.

       d. T

       e. T—The radiological prevalence of osteoarthrosis rises with age as does the radiological prevalence of cartilage calcification. Occasionally in osteoarthrosis acute episodes of inflammation may supervene and these may be due to crystals of calcium pyrophosphate.

A.8.11 a. F

       b. T—For the first three months of treatment it is recommended that a non-steroidal anti-inflammatory drug or colchicine is used concurrently.

       c. F—This may lead to attacks of acute gout when the drug is re-started leading to poor patient compliance.

       d. F

       e. T—Probenecid is a uricosuric agent and allopurinol an inhibitor of the enzyme xanthine oxidase.

Q.8.12 **Hyperuricaemia occurs in**

a. Lesch–Nyhan syndrome
b. polycythaemia rubra vera
c. primary hyperparathyroidism
d. starvation
e. thyrotoxicosis

Q.8.13 **The following statements relating to gout are correct:**

a. Males and females are almost equally affected
b. The peak age of onset is 25–35 years
c. A moderate fever may occur during the acute attack
d. The clinical severity of the attack is directly related to the serum uric acid level
e. Allopurinol acts by increasing the uric acid excretion in the urine

Q.8.14 **Calcium pyrophosphate arthropathy (pseudo-gout)**

a. is relatively common among the middle-aged and elderly
b. in its acute form, most commonly presents with shoulder pain
c. characteristically has uric acid crystals in the joint aspirate
d. radiographically shows calcification of joint cartilage
e. is controlled, as gout, by treatment with allopurinol

Q.8.15 **Secondary gout differs from the primary form in the following respects:**

a. Women are affected more frequently than in primary gout
b. A history of familial involvement is usual
c. There is a tendency towards a higher serum uric acid level and greater urinary uric acid excretion
d. There is a much higher incidence of uric acid stone formation
e. The age of onset is greater than in primary gout

For answers see over

Answers

A.8.12 a. T—The Lesch–Nyhan syndrome is an X-linked disorder associated with an over-production of urate. Subjects usually present in infancy with chorea, mental retardation and self-mutilation.

        b. T—And other myeloproliferative disorders.

        c. T

        d. T—Largely due to inhibition of renal tubular urate excretion by accumulated acids such as hydroxybutyrate formed when fat is metabolised.

        e. F—But may be found in hypothyroidism.

A.8.13 a. F—Males are more often affected than females.

        b. F—The disease is more frequently seen after the age of 40 years.

        c. T—Along with sweating, anorexia and other systemic symptoms.

        d. F

        e. F—Allopurinol inhibits the enzyme xanthine oxidase, thus preventing the conversion of xanthine and hypoxanthine to uric acid.

A.8.14 a. F—But the incidence of calcification of the articular cartilage rises with age.

        b. F—The knee and wrist are the most common sites.

        c. F—The crystals are typically of calcium pyrophosphate, i.e., rhomboidal birefringent crystals.

        d. T—This is described as chondrocalcinosis.

        e. F—Allopurinol does not benefit this condition.

A.8.15 a. F

        b. F

        c. F

        d. F

        e. T

Primary gout implies an inherited metabolic abnormality, usually unidentified. Secondary gout occurs where an identifiable, and usually acquired, cause can be found, e.g., myeloproliferative disorder, drugs, renal failure.

Q.8.16   Serum uric acid

    a. is decreased by starvation
    b. is greater in males than females
    c. is increased by treatment with steroids
    d. is decreased by oral acetylsalicylic acid at a dose of 5 g daily
    e. is increased in polycythaemia vera
    f. is decreased by treatment with colchicine

Q.8.17   Allopurinol

    a. should never be used with indomethacin
    b. may be used in renal insufficiency
    c. causes a temporary increase in serum cholesterol
    d. may precipitate gout
    e. is effective in lowering serum urate in neoplasms if used with 6-mercaptopurine.

Q.8.18   The following drugs are uricosuric agents:

    a. Probenecid
    b. Colchicine
    c. Azapropazone
    d. Allopurinol
    e. Sulphinpyrazone
    f. Hydrochlorthiazide

Q.8.19   Gout may be caused by

    a. polycythaemia rubra vera
    b. thiazide diuretics
    c. liver disease
    d. renal disease
    e. aspirin therapy
    f. all of the above

For answers see over

Answers

A.8.16 a. F—Starvation causes an increase in uric acid
          b. T
          c. F
          d. T—Aspirin is uricosuric at this dose; the cut-off is usually around 3–4 g daily.
          e. T—As a result of the increased purine turnover.
          e. F—Colchicine has no effect on serum uric acid.

A.8.17 a. F—The drugs may be successfully used in combination when allopurinol is commenced for prophylatic treatment of gout.
          b. T—Because of renal excretion, dose adjustment is necessary, otherwise toxic reactions may occur.
          c. T—Hyperlipaemia has been known to occur with this drug.
          d. T—Which is why a non-steroidal anti-inflammatory drug or colchicine must be started concurrently to cover the first two or three months of treatment.
          e. T—But caution is necessary as allopurinol prevents the metabolism of 6-mercaptopurine with resultant increasing toxicity.

A.8.18 a. T
          b. F
          c. T—And also has anti-inflammatory properties so is a useful drug in gout.
          d. F—It is a xanthine oxidase inhibitor.
          e. T
          f. F—Decreases uric acid excretion in the urine.

A.8.19 a. T—Any myeloproliferative disorder where there is a high turnover of purines may cause hyperuricaemia and gout. Indeed, gout may be the first presentation of these disorders.
          b. T—Thiazide diuretics frequently cause hyperuricaemia, although less frequently do they cause clinical gout.
          c. F
          d. T—The same considerations apply as with thiazide diuretics.
          e. T—Aspirin in doses of less than 2.4 g daily causes urate retention, whereas approaching 5–6 g daily aspirin has a uricosuric effect.
          f. F

9. Bone Disease

Q.9.1 In the following situations patients may show avascular necrosis of the bone:

a. Prolonged steroid therapy
b. Irradiation for carcinoma
c. Trauma
d. After travelling in space
e. After deep sea diving

Q.9.2 In osteomalacia

a. the condition is more common in people over 75 years old
b. males are more often affected than females
c. the housebound are more susceptible
d. long-stay patients are especially at risk
e. normal blood chemistry rules out the diagnosis

Q.9.3 The following measures are useful in the treatment of post-menopausal osteoporosis:

a. Fluoride
b. Vitamin D
c. Calcium supplements
d. Oestrogens
e. Increased physical exercise

Q.9.4 Paget's disease of bone may

a. occur in the bones of the hand
b. be extensive yet asymptomatic
c. cause hypocalcaemia
d. cause gout
e. be associated with cardiac hypertrophy

For answers see over

Answers

A.9.1 a. T
        b. T
        c. T—In particular of the hip following fractures.
        d. F—Osteoporosis is found.
        e. T—This may occur some time (up to a week) after the decompression.

A.9.2 a. T
        b. F—It is more common in females, particularly elderly females.
        c. T—Reduced mobility predisposes to osteomalacia possibly due to lack of exposure to sunlight but probably also related to poor diet.
        d. T—These patients are an extreme case and biochemical osteomalacia may be found in up to 50% of such patients.
        e. F—Serum calcium, phosphorus and alkaline phosphatase may be normal in osteomalacia. The only certain way of diagnosing this condition is by bone biopsy.

A.9.3 a. F
        b. F
        c. F
        d. T
        e. T

Although the latter two measures are of use in the treatment of post-menopausal osteoporosis, there is no evidence that they actually cause an increase in bone mass. Fluoride therapy may increase bone density in vertebrae but carries an unacceptable risk of side-effects. Vitamin D is really only of use if there is associated osteomalacia which is not uncommon in this situation. The evidence that calcium supplementation (beyond the minimum daily requirement) is useful in osteoporosis is still controversial.

A.9.4 a. T—Any bone in the body may be affected.
        b. T—The first indication may be the finding of a markedly raised alkaline phosphatase.
        c. F—Usually normocalcaemia is present
        d. F
        e. T—Due to the hyperdynamic circulatory changes in the affected bones.

Q.9.5 **The following may exacerbate post-menopausal osteoporosis in females:**

a. Lack of exercise
b. Childhood dietary deficiency of calcium
c. Corticosteroids
d. Residence in Iceland
e. Cigarette smoking

Q.9.6 **Hypophosphataemic rickets (vitamin D resistant) is characterised by**

a. autosomal recessive inheritance
b. excessive renal tubular loss of phosphate
c. short stature
d. calcification of interspinous ligaments
e. complete resistance to treatment by vitamin D

Q.9.7 **Bone scintiscanning is a useful investigation for bone disease. It is particularly helpful in**

a. osteomalacia
b. Paget's disease of bone
c. bony metastases
d. trauma
e. osteoporosis

For answers see over

Answers

A.9.5 a. T
        b. T
        c. T
        d. F
        e. T

Of all the extensive trials on post-menopausal osteoporosis, few have shown a positive benefit for calcium supplements after the menopause. There is some evidence that bone stock at the menopause may be influenced by childhood intake of calcium. Corticosteroids and cigarette smoking together with poor mobility will exacerbate the accelerated loss of bone.

A.9.6 a. F—X-linked dominant.
        b. T—Possibly also loss from the gut.
        c. T
        d. T—It may be confused with or mis-diagnosed as ankylosing spondylitis or diffuse interstitial skeletal hyperostosis.
        e. F—Treatment is with large doses of vitamin D and phosphate.

A.9.7 a. F—Osteomalacia affects the bony skeleton diffusely and there are no specific features. However pseudofractures (Looser zones) may show up as abnormally hot areas on the scan.
        b. T—There are ways of quantifying the activity of Paget's disease in terms of whole body retention of tracer and this can be used as an indication of the efficacy of treatment
        c. T—Appearances are usually diagnostic and any hot areas may be subjected to conventional radiology.
        d. T—The changes may be apparent before conventional radiographs show abnormalities.
        e. F—Unless bony collapse has occurred in, for example, an osteoporotic vertebra.

Q.9.8 **The following statements about osteomalacia in the elderly are true:**

a. In prevention the amount of sunlight received by the skin is far less important than the dietary vitamin D content
b. Low serum calcium and phosphate levels with a raised alkaline phosphatase indicate the diagnosis
c. The affected bones are not painful unless fractured
d. Bony deformity is rare
e. With an unco-operative patient, a single dose of vitamin D can be effective treatment.

Q.9.9 **In Paget's disease**

a. the skull is most commonly affected
b. the extent of the disease is readily ascertained by the radioactive uptake of the lesions on bone scintiscanning
c. the best measure of disease activity is the serum alkaline phosphatase level
d. painful lesions are an indication for active treatment
e. calcitonin should be administered daily

Q.9.10 **Paget's disease may be treated with oral disodium etidronate. The effects of this drug in Paget's disease include**

a. a decrease in bone pain
b. an improvement in bone deformity
c. an increase in urinary hydroxyproline excretion
d. an improvement in symptoms due to nerve root compression
e. a decrease in the incidence of bone tumour

For answers see over

Answers

A.9.8 a. F—Plasma levels of vitamin D in old people are closely related to their exposure to sunlight during the summer months.
  b. T—Preferably supported by the characteristic histopathology revealed by bone biopsy.
  c. F—This statement is true of senile osteoporosis. Bone pain and tenderness are characteristic of osteomalacia.
  d. T—Unlike osteomalacia in children (rickets).
  e. T—A single intramuscular or oral dose of vitamin D is probably sufficient. A typical dose is 300 000 ɪu.

A.9.9 a. F—The axial skeleton and weight-bearing bones are more often affected.
  b. T—Paget's disease is readily demonstrated by bone-seeking radioisotopes which are adsorbed onto hydroxyapatite.
  c. T—The urinary hydroxyproline excretion is another index of activity.
  d. T—If the disease is known to be active and the pain has not responded readily to analgesics, anti-Pagetic treatment is indicated.
  e. F—Although, occasionally, daily administration may be needed, the usual regime is to start treatment with three times weekly subcutaneous injections of calcitonin.

A.9.10 a. T
  b. F
  c. F—Urinary hydroxyproline is increased in Paget's disease due to the high bone turnover. Successful treatment with etidronate causes a decrease in the 24-hour excretion.
  d. T
  e. F—There is no evidence that any treatment for Paget's disease decreases the ultimate risk of osteosarcoma.

Q.9.11   Osteomalacia

a. is due to a failure in development of osteoid
b. causes bone pain
c. is rarely associated with muscle weakness
d. may be associated with a positive Trousseau's sign
e. is caused by treatment with phenytoin and responds to thera-peutic doses of vitamin D

Q.9.12   Diffuse idiopathic skeletal hyperostosis (DISH or Forestier's disease)

a. is seen more frequently in patients with diabetes mellitus
b. may be confused with ankylosing spondylitis
c. may be caused by treatment with etretinate
d. is associated with raised parathormone levels
e. is associated with plantar pustulosis (pustulotic arthro-osteitis)

Q.9.13   In a male aged 70 years with low back pain and an elevated alkaline phosphatase, the following diagnoses are possible:

a. Senile osteoporosis
b. Osteomalacia
c. Myeloma
d. Paget's disease
e. Secondaries from carcinoma of prostate

For answers see over

Answers

A.9.11 a. F—An over-production of uncalcified osteoid is the histological hallmark of this condition.

b. T

c. F—Proximal muscle weakness frequently occurs.

d. T—In association with hypocalcaemia, Chvostek's sign may also be present.

e. T—Although large doses of vitamin D may be needed initially to correct the deficiency. Following initial treatment small doses of vitamin D are necessary indefinitely. Clinical vitamin D deficiency occurs in phenytoin therapy as a result of hepatic enzyme induction.

A.9.12 a. T—As is capsulitis of the shoulder.

b. T—Pain and stiffness in the back, although the symptoms are rarely as severe as in ankylosing spondylitis.

c. T—And since this drug is given for psoriasis, confusion may arise as to the presence of spondylitic changes with the psoriasis.

d. F—No biochemical abnormality.

e. F—Pustulotic arthro-osteitis is probably a variant of psoriatic arthropathy that may be associated with sacroiliitis and, in particular, an arthritis of the sternoclavicular and manubriosternal joints.

A.9.13 a. F

b. T

c. T

d. T

e. T

In senile osteoporosis, alkaline phosphatase is invariably normal unless a crush fracture has occurred when there may be transient slight elevation in the alkaline phosphatase. Osteomalacia occurs commonly in elderly in-patient populations but the prevalence in the community is less certain.

10. *Miscellaneous Questions*

Questions

Q.10.1 **The following are synovial joints:**

a. Symphysis pubis
b. Sacroiliac joint
c. Sacrococcygeal joint
d. Lumbo-sacral joint
e. Patellofemoral joint

Q.10.2 **The following features of Marfan's syndrome distinguish it from homocystinuria:**

a. Autosomal dominant inheritance
b. Lens dislocation
c. Joint laxity
d. Aortic rupture
e. Arachnodactyly

Q.10.3 **Match the following:**

a. Increase in glove size
b. Increase in hat size
c. Decrease in size of spoon which can be used to eat soup
d. Inability to keep spectacles on the nose
e. Loss of ability to see straight ahead

A. Scleroderma
B. Relapsing polychondritis
C. Acromegaly
D. Ankylosing spondylitis
E. Paget's disease of bone

Q.10.4 **A 16-year-old female presents with a two-year history of painful swollen knees. On examination she has generalised hyperlaxity marked at the knee joints. You would advise the following management strategies:**

a. Calipers for both knee joints to prevent hyperextension
b. Resting splints for both knees
c. Quadriceps, hamstring and calf muscle exercises
d. Regular review with the advice that as she grows older the joint hyperlaxity is likely to disappear
e. Intra-articular steroid injections for both knees

For answers see over

Answers

A.10.1 a. F—This is a cartilaginous joint.
        b. T—Although the amount of movement is extremely limited.
        c. F—This is an intervertebral joint.
        d. F—Also an intervertebral joint.
        e. T

A.10.2 a. T
        b. F
        c. T
        d. T
        e. F

Homocystinuria may appear clinically similar to Marfan's syndrome but it is subject to autosomal recessive inheritance. Diagnosis may be made by obtaining a positive cyanide–nitroprusside test on urine.

A.10.3 a. C
        b. E
        c. A
        d. B
        e. D

A.10.4 a. F—Although this may seem like an extreme measure, very occasionally in severe cases such calipers are necessary to prevent damage and premature osteoarthritis to the joints.
        b. F—These will have no effect since this is not an inflammatory arthritis.
        c. T—Improving muscle tone and strength will "stiffen" the knee and help prevent the hyperextension that occurs on walking.
        d. T—Although not everyone is happy with this advice.
        e. F—Although a chronic low grade synovitis may occur in hyperlaxity, this is a secondary event. Theoretically, intra-articular steroids may accelerate any damage due to hyperextension of the joint.

Q.10.5 **In the following conditions hypermobile joints may be found:**

a. Marfan's syndrome
b. Osteogenesis imperfecta
c. Hyperthyroidism
d. Hypertelorism
e. Ehlers–Danlos syndrome

Q.10.6 **The following diseases may cause a haemarthrosis of the knee joint:**

a. Pigmented villonodular synovitis
b. Henoch–Schönlein purpura
c. Rheumatoid arthritis
d. Torn medial meniscus
e. Factor IX deficiency (Christmas disease)

Q.10.7 **A male aged 25 years presents with an acutely painful swollen knee. The following clinical features may help in establishing a diagnosis:**

a. Employment as a carpet fitter
b. Consumption of 5 pints of beer daily
c. Coincidental Achilles tendinitis
d. A history of conjuctivitis
e. Recent (within 5 days) mushroom ingestion

For answers see over

Answers

A.10.5 a. T
        b. T
        c. F
        d. F
        e. T

Hypermobile or hyperlax joints are commonly seen in females under the age of 20 years and some figures have quoted a prevalence of 15% in this group. Whether the idiopathic cases are due to an abnormality in collagen or in muscle tone is still not clear. However, congenital collagen abnormalities such as occur in Marfan's syndrome, osteogenesis imperfecta and Ehlers–Danlos syndrome may also cause hyperlaxity, as may widespread muscle hypotonia.

A.10.6 a. T—Pigmented villonodular synovitis frequently causes a symmetrical erosive arthritis of the knees, the characteristic of which is blood-stained aspirate and haemosiderin pigmentation with giant cells in the synovial histology.
        b. F—A monarthritis with a clear effusion may be found.
        c. F—Often the effusion appears yellow-green in colour.
        d. F—Since the cartilage is avascular; although, if other structures are injured at the same time, such as the tibial plateau, or a synovial tear occurs, a haemarthrosis may occur.
        e. T

A.10.7 a. T—Carpet fitters are required to kneel a lot and use a tool known as a stretcher by which the carpet is fitted neatly to the walls. This requires them to repeatedly hammer their knee against a padded handle, thus precipitating prepatella bursitis (housemaid's knee).
        b. T—Heavy alcohol ingestion may cause hyperuricaemia and clinical gout manifest as acute bursitis or synovitis.
        c. T—An enthesitis would suggest Reiter's syndrome or another of the group of seronegative spondarthritides.
        d. T—Although conjuctivitis is a relatively common disorder and caution would be needed in interpreting this part of the history.
        e. F

Q.10.8   **The following diseases may cause a symmetrical arthropathy:**

  a. Gout
  b. Rheumatoid arthritis
  c. Tertiary syphilis
  d. Gonorrhoea
  e. Congenital syphilis
  f. Tuberculosis

Q.10.9   **Raynaud's phenomenon**

  a. is pain in the fingers on exposure to cold
  b. may cause gangrene of the digits
  c. may be the first indication of a connective tissue disorder
  d. is a feature of Marfan's syndrome
  e. is frequently seen in people who work with vibrating tools

Q.10.10   **The ulnar nerve**

  a. carries fibres from the C6 nerve root
  b. supplies the muscles of the outer half of the thenar eminence
  c. supplies adductor pollicis
  d. when damaged at the elbow, produces wrist drop
  e. may be trapped in the carpal tunnel

For answers see over

Answers

A.10.8 a. F—Attacks of gout or acute podagra classically affect the first MTP joints but may occur elsewhere. Chronic tophaceous gout may mimic asymmetrical polyarthropathy.

b. T

c. F—Charcot joints resulting from Tabes dorsalis are usually asymmetrical.

d. F—Usually an asymmetrical septic arthritis.

e. T—Clutton's joints are often symmetrical, for example, at the knees.

f. F—This usually produces a large joint monarthritis.

A.10.9 a. F—Raynaud's phenomenon is frequently mis-diagnosed historically. The classical description is of marked change in colour of the fingers on exposure to cold so that part of the fingers turn white. Depending upon the ambient temperature this phase of ischaemia may itself be painful. When blood returns to the ischaemic area further pain is produced.

b. T—During a prolonged period of vasospasm.

c. T—Although probably the commonest diagnostic label attached to Raynaud's phenomenon is idiopathic.

d. F

e. T—Otherwise known as vibration-white finger and now classified as a pensionable industrial disease.

A.10.10 a. F—Carries fibres from C8, T1 and occasionally C7.

b. F—These are supplied by the median nerve.

c. T

d. F—Damage to the radial nerve produces wrist drop.

e. F

Questions

Q.10.11 Clubbing

    a. may be a manifestation of a congenital defect in connective tissue

    b. may be associated with a painful arthropathy

    c. is caused by a humoral factor normally inactivated by the lungs

    d. is evident radiologically

    e. occurs more often in the hands than the feet

    f. may be caused by hyperthyroidism

Q.10.12 The following diseases may cause pain and swelling in the joints:

    a. Primary idiopathic thrombocytopenic purpura

    b. Classical haemophilia (Factor VIII deficiency)

    c. Monocytic leukaemia

    d. Henoch–Schönlein purpura

    e. Polycythaemia rubra vera

Q.10.13 A 30-year-old guitar playing busker complains that he cannot perform for more than one hour due to weakness of his left hand. Further questioning reveals that he occasionally experiences mild paraesthesiae of the thumb and forefinger of both hands. Examination reveals bilateral wasting of the thenar eminence. Nerve conduction tests across the wrists give the following results:

		Right	Left
Motor latency (milliseconds)	Median nerve	5	8
	Ulnar nerve	3	2.5
Sensory amplitude	Median nerve	10	5
(microvolts)	Ulnar nerve	12	13

The history, clinical findings and investigations are compatible with:

    a. Left carpal tunnel syndrome only

    b. Bilateral carpal tunnel syndrome

    c. Peripheral neuropathy

    d. Cervical syringomyelia

    e. Over-use syndrome (repetitive strain injury)

For answers see over

Answers

A.10.11 a. T—Pachydermoperiostitis.
b. T—Periostitis at the wrists (hypertrophic pulmonary osteoarthropathy) may be mistaken for an arthritis at the wrist but in
addition true synovitis may be found at other joints.
c. T—There is some debate about this at the moment. A neural
mechanism has been implicated since clubbing may disappear
following vagotomy but recent evidence (J Rheum (1987) 14:
6–7) suggested that a humoral factor normally inactivated by
the lungs may cause the clubbing. This humoral factor may be
over-produced in conditions of the bowel such as carcinoid
syndrome.
d. T—Tufting may be evident in the terminal phalanges.
e. F
f. T—Also known as thyroid acropachy.

A.10.12 a. F
b. T
c. T
d. T
e. T

It is worth noting that any disease involving a high turnover of
nucleic acids, and in particular any myeloproliferative disorder,
may cause hyperuricaemia and episodes of acute gout.

A.10.13 a. F
b. T—The motor latency of the median nerve in both hands is
delayed, more so on the left. Depending on the placement of
the electrodes the latency is usually less than 4.5 milliseconds.
Nerve conduction tests can be normal with symptoms of
carpal tunnel syndrome but usually if wasting is evident there
are objective changes on electrophysiological testing.
c. F—This is excluded because of the normal motor conduction
in the ulnar nerve and normal sensory amplitude in the ulnar
nerve (usually regarded as normal if above 10 microvolts).
d. F—Peripheral nerve conduction would be normal with evidence of denervation on EMG.
e. F—There are no neurophysiological abnormalities in this
condition.

Q.10.14 **The figure represents the result of an ischaemic lactate test. The following statements are true:**

a. The test is normal
b. The result indicates McArdle's disease
c. The patient must be on a fat-free diet for one week before this test
d. In a patient with exercise-induced muscle pain and fatiguability, the test excludes a significant metabolic problem

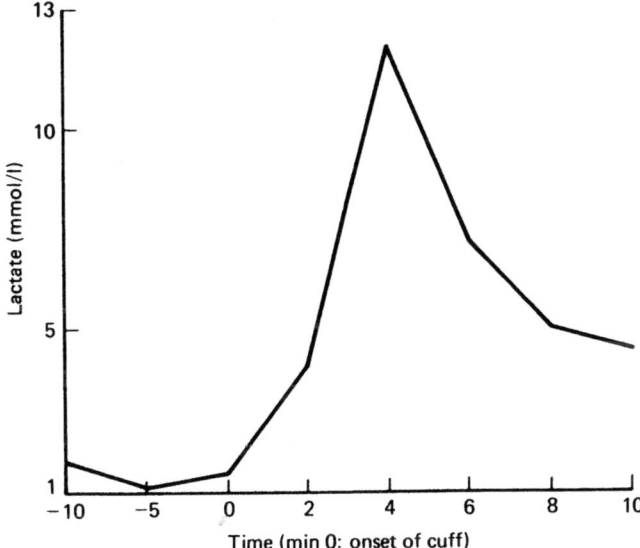

Q.10.15 **In Charcot joints**

a. joint subluxation is often found
b. intra-articular fractures are common
c. cartilage destruction and hypertrophic bone formation are marked
d. bony ankylosis is common
e. the joint may be painful

For answers see over

Answers

A.10.14 a. T—A normal individual will show a threefold rise in lactate four minutes after the start of occlusion of the blood pressure to the arm.

        b. F—In McArdle's disease, where there is a deficiency in phosphorylase, patients are unable to release glucose from muscle glycogen and hence do not produce lactate by anaerobic metabolism.

        c. F—The only stipulation is that patients are fasting for four hours before a test.

        d. F—Other rare enzymatic deficiencies such as acid maltase produce a normal ischaemic lactate test and diagnosis is by enzyme assay on muscle tissue.

A.10.15 a. T
        b. T
        c. T
        d. F
        e. T

The commonest causes of Charcot joints are diabetes mellitus and neurological disease (such as syringomyelia) but syphilitic Charcot joints are still seen. Typically, they show gross disorganisation, subluxation and new bone formation. Paradoxically, these joints may occasionally be painful, although the degree of pain is not as severe as would be expected from the radiological and clinical appearance of the joint.

Q.10.16 **In Whipple's disease**

    a. malabsorption may occur
    b. skin pigmentation occurs
    c. joint symptoms may precede other symptoms by many years
    d. lymphadenopathy and polyserositis may occur
    e. bacterial cell wall fragments have been found in synovial membrane

Q.10.17 **A male aged 22 years presents with a painful swollen knee joint. Haematological investigation reveals a Hb 10.4 g/dl, normal platelet count, normal prothrombin time, normal bleeding time but prolonged activated partial thromboplastin time. The following haematological disorders may cause these findings:**

    a. Henoch–Schönlein purpura
    b. Factor IX deficiency (Christmas disease)
    c. Factor VIII deficiency (classical haemophilia)
    d. von Willebrand's disease
    e. Factor VII deficiency

Q.10.18 **In osteochondritis dissecans**

    a. the knee joint is most frequently involved
    b. intermittent mechanical locking of the knee is characteristic
    c. prognosis is better in children
    d. the condition is always unilateral
    e. a positive family history is sometimes obtained

For answers see over

Answers

A.10.16 a. T
           b. T
           c. T
           d. T
           e. F

Whipple's disease is characterised by a migratory polyarthritis associated with malabsorption. A characteristic finding is that of PAS-staining granules in macrophages in the intestinal mucosa. Furthermore, rod-shaped organisms have been demonstrated in the lamina propria of the intestinal mucosa but not in the synovial membrane. Prolonged treatment with antibiotics produces clinical improvement of the arthritis and eliminates these rod-shaped organisms.

A.10.17 a. F
           b. T
           c. T
           d. F
           e. F

Henoch-Schönlein purpura is not associated with a clotting defect nor is von Willebrand's disease. With Factor VII deficiency, the prothrombin time would be prolonged.

A.10.18 a. T—The ankle and hip may also be involved.
           b. T—Following locking an effusion may develop.
           c. T—Occasionally fragments may reunite in children.
           d. F—The condition is frequently bilateral.
           e. T

Treatment is expectant. Large fragments have been pinned in their existing position but smaller fragments are removed when they become detached. The condition predisposes to osteoarthrosis.

Q.10.19 The following are features of Marfan's syndrome:

   a. Dislocation of the lens
   b. Scoliosis
   c. Autosomal recessive inheritance
   d. Mitral regurgitation
   e. Painful joints

Q.10.20 You aspirate synovial fluid from a joint. The laboratory results are: cell count, 160 000/cu mm; cell type, 90% neutrophil; glucose, 0.5 mmol/l. The following diagnoses are compatible:

   a. Osteoarthritis
   b. Septic arthritis
   c. Rheumatoid arthritis
   d. Acute gout
   e. Pigmented villonodular synovitis

Q.10.21 You would advise against sunbathing in a patient with

   a. psoriatic arthritis
   b. rheumatoid arthritis
   c. systemic lupus erythematosus
   d. acute intermittent porphyria
   e. porphyria cutanea larda
   f. sarcoidosis

For answers see over

Answers

A.10.19
a. T
b. T—Associated with joint laxity and kyphosis.
c. F—Autosomal dominant.
d. T—And aortic dilatation, although rarely.
e. T—Possibly associated with hypermobility.

A.10.20
a. F—Cell counts rarely exceed 15 000.
b. T
c. F—Cell counts rarely exceed 100 000.
d. F—Although cell counts may exceed 100 000 and consist mainly of neutrophils, glucose levels, although modestly decreased, are never markedly diminished. A markedly diminished glucose in synovial fluid is usually due to septic arthritis or to tuberculous infection.
e. F—Usually a haemarthrosis is obtained in this condition.

A.10.21
a. F—Sunlight is often beneficial to psoriasis and the joint disease may parallel the severity in skin inflammation.
b. F—Unless the patient is being treated with anti-malarials which can cause photosensitivity (occasionally NSAIDs cause a photosensitive rash).
c. T—Photosensitive rashes are common.
d. F—The cutaneous manifestations of the other porphyrias are not apparent in classical acute intermittent porphyria.
e. T—Usually sunbathing causes a blistering rash leaving hyper-pigmented scars.
f. F—Erythema nodosum and lupus pernio may occur in sarcoidosis although neither are exacerbated by sunlight.

Q.10.22 **Arthritis mutilans occurs in the following conditions:**

    a. Rheumatoid arthritis
    b. Reiter's syndrome
    c. Gout
    d. Psoriatic arthritis
    e. Whipple's disease
    f. All of the above

Q.10.23 **The following are true statements:**

    a. Gout is confirmed by the presence of a high serum uric acid
    b. Severe osteoarthritis of the hip is invariably evident clinically
    c. In a young male with chronic low back pain the presence of HLA-B27 confirms the diagnosis of ankylosing spondylitis
    d. The symptom of early morning stiffness of the joints suggests a diagnosis of rheumatoid arthritis
    e. Normal nerve conduction tests exclude a diagnosis of carpal tunnel syndrome

Q.10.24 **Raynaud's phenomenon may be the prodrome of**

    a. rheumatoid arthritis
    b. eosinophilic fasciitis
    c. scleroderma
    d. systemic lupus erythematosus
    e. carcinoid syndrome

For answers see over

Answers

A.10.22 a. T
b. F—Reiter's classically affects the larger joints such as the wrist, knee, ankle and tarsal joints.
c. F—Although chronic tophaceous gout may produce severe deformity of the fingers.
d. T—Together with rheumatoid arthritis, the commonest causes.
e. F—Usually causes an intermittent transitory synovitis of large joints.
f. F

A.10.23 a. F—Gout is confirmed by the presence of uric acid crystals in fluid aspirated from the joint.
b. T—This may not be so with rheumatoid arthritis.
c. F—Although 90% of cases of ankylosing spondylitis carry the HLA-B27 antigen, further evidence is required to make a firm diagnosis, otherwise we are in danger of encouraging a cohort of B27-positive low-back-pain invalids.
d. F—Early morning stiffness may also occur in osteoarthritis though usually it is less severe and of shorter duration.
e. F—The intermittent nature of this syndrome, especially in the early stages, may fail to provide the confirmation required on nerve conduction tests. Some rheumatologists use an injection of steroid into the carpal tunnel as a diagnostic test.

A.10.24 a. T
b. F—Although this disease is classified with the scleroderma group, Raynaud's phenomenon is not a feature.
c. T
d. T
e. F

Q.10.25 **Match the following:**

Nerve root irritation

a. L3
b. L4
c. L5
d. S1
e. S2

Clinical sequelae

A. Anaesthesia of the sole of the foot
B. Weakness of dorsiflexion of the foot
C. Wasting of the buttock
D. Weakness of hip abduction
E. Pain in the knee

Q.10.26 **Match the following:**

Nerve root irritation

a. C4
b. C5
c. C6
d. C7
e. C8
f. T1

Clinical sequelae

A. Loss of biceps reflex
B. Pain in the shoulder
C. Wasting of the interossei muscles
D. Weakness of wrist extension
E. Anaesthesia over the medial epicondyle of the elbow
F. Weakness of wrist flexion

For answers see over

Answers

A.10.25   a. E
              b. B
              c. D
              d. A
              e. C

A.10.26   a. B
              b. A
              c. D
              d. F
              e. C
              f. E

Q.10.27 **The following eponymous statements are true:**

    a. Finkelstein's sign is pain at the base of the thumb when this digit is fully flexed and the wrist passively moved into full ulnar deviation

    b. Phalen's test is positive if parasthesiae are produced in the thumb and index finger when the wrist is passively extended for 60 seconds

    c. Atlanto-axial subluxation may cause a positive Hoffman's sign

    d. The Trendelenberg test is positive when the contralateral hip sags as the patient stands on the ipsilateral leg

    e. Patients who can touch their toes are likely to have a normal Schober's test

    f. Kellgren's sign is elicitable in the knee

Q.10.28 **Dupuytren's contracture**

    a. may be associated with sexual dysfunction in the male

    b. affects both sexes equally

    c. may be associated with plantar fibromatosis

    d. is found more frequently in patients with idiopathic epilepsy

    e. in the early stages, responds to treatment with oral steroids

Q.10.29 **Familial Mediterranean Fever**

    a. occurs solely in ethnic groups around the Mediterranean

    b. is characterised by polyserositis

    c. often causes a chronic arthritis

    d. is characterised by autosomal dominant inheritance

    e. may be complicated at a relatively early age by systemic amyloidosis

For answers see over

Answers

A.10.27 a. T
  b. F—When the wrist is flexed for 60 seconds.
  c. T
  d. T
  e. F—The lumbar spine may be fused with all the movement taking place at the hips.
  f. T—This is a sign for minimal effusion at the knee. The fluid can be passed back and forth from medial to lateral compartments by gentle stroking at each side of the knee.

A.10.28 a. T—Peyronie's syndrome is associated with it.
  b. F—Males are more affected than females in the ratio of 6:1.
  c. T
  d. T
  e. F—The only successful treatment is surgery.

A.10.29 a. F—It may also occur in Arabs, Jews and Armenians.
  b. T
  c. F—Usually a transient oligoarthritis lasting about a week occurs. Very occasionally a chronic arthritis is found.
  d. F—Autosomal recessive.
  e. T—And this may be prevented by treatment with colchicine.

Familial Mediterranean Fever may mimic juvenile chronic arthritis, SLE, primary Sjögren's syndrome or a seronegative arthropathy and should be considered where seronegative oligoarthritis occurs with fever and serositis in patients from the Mediterranean littoral and other Middle Eastern countries.

11. *Rehabilitation and Surgery*

Q.11.1 **Maintenance of independent mobility is an important aim in chronic rheumatic disease. The following statements are true:**

a. In ankylosing spondylitis patients without rotatory movement of the cervical spine should not drive a car
b. Patients considered unfit to drive a car should be referred directly to the Driver and Vehicle Licencing Centre (DVLC)
c. A patient with juvenile chronic arthritis may obtain a driving licence at the age of 16 years
d. A rigid cervical collar is recommended for patients who have atlanto-axial subluxation
e. Any necessary modifications to the car are provided free of charge

Q.11.2 **In the UK the mobility allowance**

a. is a tax-free, weekly cash benefit
b. is payable only on the recommendation of a hospital specialist
c. is subject to strict objective eligibility criteria
d. may be used to buy an outdoor electric wheelchair
e. is only payable to those capable of driving a car

Q.11.3 **A married 70-year-old female with chronic rheumatoid arthritis has mobility difficulties due to lower limb joint destruction. The following statements are true:**

a. She may be eligible for mobility allowance
b. Disabled car stickers are only available on the recommendation of a hospital specialist
c. Her husband may be eligible for an attendance allowance
d. Stairlifts are provided by Social Services
e. A wheelchair may be provided by the local Occupational Therapy Department

For answers see over

Answers

A.11.1
a. F—In order to maintain their driving ability, wide panoramic rear view mirrors and adequate side mirrors are necessary.

b. F—The onus is on the patient to inform the DVLC of any disability. The doctor should recommend the patient to do this but only in exceptional circumstances should the doctor write to the DVLC direct.

c. T—If they are in receipt of a mobility allowance.

d. T—And, in addition, head-rest supports are recommended in this group of patients and in patients with ankylosing spondylitis, to guard against whiplash injury.

e. F—Although they may be provided under the Motability scheme or out of the mobility allowance.

A.11.2
a. T

b. F—Anyone may apply for a mobility allowance and assessment is made by a locally appointed doctor, usually a general practitioner.

c. F—The eligibility criteria are somewhat ill-defined although the regulations state the patient must be unable, or virtually unable, to walk.

d. T

e. F—However, patients who are comatose or otherwise unable to travel in a car are not eligible.

A.11.3
a. F—Patients are only eligible for mobility allowance if they apply before the age of 65 years.

b. F—Disabled car stickers may be provided with the signature of any doctor.

c. F—Attendance allowance is only payable to the person requiring assistance. Although the eligibility is ill-defined, normally the person applying must need help in self-care.

d. T

e. F—Wheelchairs are provided on prescription by the local Appliance and Limb Fitting Centre on the recommendation of any doctor.

Q.11.4 The following may be useful to a patient with severe osteoarthritis of the knee in order tó maintain his independence:

a. A wheelchair
b. Elevation of the toilet seat
c. Reduction in the height of the bed
d. A knee brace for fixed varus deformity
e. Regular attendance at the local physiotherapy department

Q.11.5 Walking sticks

a. should be used on the opposite side to the affected joint
b. may reduce the load in a weight-bearing joint by some 50%
c. may cause premature osteoarthritis of the wrist
d. are of little use in rheumatoid arthritis where severe deformity of the metacarpophalangeal joints has occurred
e. need little maintenance

Q.11.6 Physical methods of treatment are frequently used in conjunction with pharmacological measures. The following statements are true:

a. Shortwave diathermy is hazardous after joint replacement
b. Cardiac pacemakers may present a hazard
c. Cervical manipulation is contraindicated in subjects on anticoagulants
d. Spinal exercises are contraindicated in ankylosing spondylitis
e. Hydrotherapy is contraindicated in the presence of chronic obstructive airways disease

For answers see over

Answers

A.11.4 a. F—It is important to assess a patient for surgery prior to ordering a wheelchair. It is much easier to rehabilitate a patient following surgery if he is ambulatory using a stick or frame prior to the operation.

          b. T—This may be provided by Social Services.

          c. F—If the bed is too low the patient may be unable to get up in the morning.

          d. F—A knee brace is unlikely to help fixed deformity. Only when the deformity becomes apparent on weight bearing will a brace be of use.

          e. F—The effort involved in attending the local department may be counter-productive. A more reasonable approach is to recommend and teach exercises to be performed at home although regular review is necessary in order to ensure they are carried out.

A.11.5 a. T

          b. T

          c. F

          d. F—Moulded, large-handled walking sticks may be provided.

          e. F—Attention must be paid to the handle and ferrule, which needs changing regularly.

A.11.6 a. T—Because the metal concentrates the emission.

          b. T—These may be affected by high frequency radiation from some machines.

          c. T

          d. F—Just the contrary.

          e. T—Although this rule should not be applied rigidly and depends on the exercise tolerance of the individual patient.

Q.11.7 **The following statements are correct. In rheumatoid arthritis:**

    a. Wearing a reinforced low lumbar support reduces episodes of low back pain

    b. In atlantoaxial subluxation it is advisable to wear a soft cervical collar at all times

    c. Rest splints reduce joint pain and help prevent deformity

    d. Patients are often unable to apply splints because of existing functional problems

    e. Subtalar deformities invariably need correction by means of a side caliper

Q.11.8 **The following are indications to refer a patient with low back pain for surgery:**

    a. Recent urinary difficulties

    b. Increasing rest pain

    c. Sciatica

    d. Increasing weakness of plantar flexion of the ankle with wasting of the calf

    e. Global sensory loss

Q.11.9 **You have been asked about the possibility of total hip replacement for a 75-year-old arthritic female. The following statements are true:**

    a. The usual disease necessitating total hip replacement is osteoarthritis

    b. The predominant indication for surgery is the relief of pain

    c. Patients over 75 years are usually unacceptable for operation

    d. If a urinary tract infection is present it must be eradicated before surgery

    e. One must always warn the patient that revision surgery to replace the artificial hip joint is more or less inevitable after five years

For answers see over

Answers

A.11.7 a. F—There is no evidence that wearing a support of this kind reduces episodes of low back pain in either rheumatoid arthritis or degenerative spinal disease.

        b. F—Providing no neurological symptoms or signs are present, then it is only recommended that a collar is worn when in situations at risk such as riding in a car. In this case the collar should be of the rigid variety. In atlantoaxial subluxation with neurological symptoms or signs, improvement may be obtained by the use of a rigid day collar and a soft night collar. Nevertheless, if symptoms or signs progress surgical advice should be sought.

        c. T

        d. T—Up to 50% of prescribed splints (including footwear) are not used.

        e. F—Subtalar deformities may be corrected by use of modelled insoles, external modification of the footwear with built-up and splayed heels, and cosmetic calipers fitted inside the shoe.

A.11.8 a. T
        b. F
        c. F
        d. T
        e. F

The indications for surgical intervention vary from surgeon to surgeon but the only clear indications are increasing and objective neurological deficit or sphincter disturbance together with a radiologically demonstrable, and surgically treatable, lesion.

A.11.9 a. T—Idiopathic osteoarthritis is the commonest reason.

        b. T—Stiffness and immobility may be improved by surgery but the operation excels at pain relief.

        c. F—Age itself is no contra-indication, but the patient must be sufficiently healthy to survive the operation and benefit from the result.

        d. T—This, and any other focus of infection, should be eliminated because of the danger of sepsis.

        e. F—A well-performed Charnley total hip replacement will usually last for 10 years or more depending on the use.

Q.11.10 **The following are reasonable surgical procedures in musculoskeletal disease:**

    a. Laminectomy in ankylosing spondylitis

    b. Excision arthoplasty of the metatarsal heads in rheumatoid arthritis where metatarsalgia occurs due to subluxation of the metatarsophalangeal joints

    c. Synovectomy of the knee in early rheumatoid arthritis

    d. Fusion of the atlanto-axial joint due to subluxation in rheumatoid arthritis

    e. Osteotomy for varus deformity of the knee joint in osteoarthritis

Q.11.11 **In rheumatoid arthritis the following conditions need surgical attention:**

    a. Ruptured long head of biceps

    b. Ruptured extensor communis tendon of hand

    c. "Trigger finger"

    d. "Mallet finger"

    e. Carpal tunnel syndrome

For answers see over

Answers

A.11.10 a. F—Ankylosing spondylitis frequently presents with sciatic-like pain and although other features of ankylosing spondylitis are present, laminectomy may be performed. A consequence of the immobilisation following surgery is increased stiffness of the spine.

          b. T

          c. F—Conservative treatment for synovial inflammation should be tried first, including systemic therapy with disease-modifying drugs and local therapy with intra-articular steroids. Synovectomy is a disappointing operation in that regrowth of the excised tissue may occur; about a third benefit from the operation.

          d. F—Fusion of the atlanto-axial joint is a hazardous operation and should only be undertaken for severe and progressing neurological signs associated with myelographic or CT evidence of cord compression.

          e. T

A.11.11 a. F—Surgical treatment is unnecessary and often the patient presents far too late for repair. The long head of biceps is not absolutely essential and many of its actions can be taken over by bracho-radialis.

          b. T—This is a simple operation often not requiring tendon transfer or graft.

          c. F—This complication can be treated by an injection of hydrocortisone into the affected area where proliferating rheumatoid synovium causes a stenosis in the flexor tendon sheath. Occasionally surgical treatment is necessary.

          d. F—Splintage is all that is necessary.

          e. F—Providing symptoms and signs are not severe, this can also be readily treated by local injection of corticosteroid into the carpal tunnel. The indications for surgical intervention are (i) poor response to injection therapy and (ii) muscle wasting. It is important to note that as the disease remits this complication may also remit.